PAEDIATRIC
DENTISTRY FAQ
ALPHA DENTISTRY vol. 3
ASSEMBLED EDITION

by ACHIEVER OF THE YEAR LINKEDIN AND TOWN HALL
EY NOMINEE ENTREPRENEUR OF THE YEAR
GRAND HOMAGE LYS DIVERSITY
WORLD'S TOP100 DOCTORS
CREA GLOBAL AWARD
Dr. BAK NGUYEN, DMD, FORCES

&

USA PAEDIATRIC DENTISTS

Dr. PAUL DOMINIQUE, DMD, MS, PEDODONTIST
Dr. RICHARD SIMPSON, DMD, PEDODONTIST
Dr. MARILYN SANDOR, DDS, MS, PEDODONTIST
Dr. NIDHI TANEJA, DDS, MSD, PEDODONTIST

INTERNATIONAL PAEDIATRIC DENTISTS

Dr. AURORA ALVA, DMD, PEDODONTIST
Dr. NOUR AMMAR, BDS, MS, PEDODONTIST
Dr. AILÍN CABRERA-MATTA, DMD, MS, Ph.D. PEDODONTIST
Dr. PIERLUIGI PELAGALLI, DDS, PEDODONTIST
Dr. PRRIYA PORWAL, BDS, MSD, PEDODONTIST

BY ALPHA DENTISTS TO EVERYONE IN THE WORLD SEEKING ANSWERS ON THEIR QUEST FOR A BETTER ORAL HEALTH AND SMILE.

by Dr. BAK NGUYEN

ISBN: 978-1-998750-18-4

Published by: Dr. BAK PUBLISHING COMPANY
Dr.BAK 0132

DISCLAIMER

ABOUT THE AUTHORS

From Canada 🍁, **Dr. BAK NGUYEN**, Nominee Ernst and Young Entrepreneur of the year, Grand Homage Lys DIVERSITY, LinkedIn & TownHall Achiever of the year and TOP 100 Doctors 2021. In 2023, he made the CREA GLOBAL AWARD list. Dr. Bak is a cosmetic dentist, CEO and founder of Mdex & Co. His company is revolutionizing the dental field.

Speaker and motivator, he holds the world record of writing 120 books in 5 years accumulating many world records (to be officialized). Before that, he held the world record of writing 9 books over 12 months, then, 15 books within 15 months to set the bar even higher with the world record of 36 books written within 18 months + 1 week.

By his second author anniversary, he scored his new landmark world record of 48 books within 24 months. And then 72 books in 36 months. By the 4th anniversary, Dr. Bak scored his usual landmark of writing 96 books over 48 months, but he pushed even further, scoring also the landmark world record of 100 books written within 4 years and then, 120 books written in 5 years! His books are covering:

ENTREPRENEURSHIP - LEADERSHIP - QUEST OF IDENTITY - DENTISTRY AND MEDICINE - PARENTING - CHILDREN BOOKS - PHILOSOPHY

In 2003, he founded Mdex, a dental company upon which in 2018, he launched the most ambitious private endeavour to reform the dental industry, Canada-wide. Philosopher, he has close to his heart the quest of happiness of the people surrounding him, patients and colleagues alike. In 2020, he launched an International collaborative initiative named **THE ALPHAS** to share knowledge and for Entrepreneurs and Doctors to thrive through the Greatest Pandemic and Economic depression of our time.

In 2016, he co-found with Tranie Vo, Emotive World Incorporated, a tech research company to use technology to empower happiness and sharing. U.A.X. the ultimate audio experience is the landmark project on which the team is advancing, utilizing the technics of the movie industry and the advancement in ARTIFICIAL INTELLIGENCE to save the book industry and upgrade the continuing education space.

These projects have allowed Dr. Nguyen to attract interest from the international and diplomatic community and he is now the centre of a global discussion on the wellbeing and the future of the health profession. It is in that matter that he shares his thoughts and encourages the health community to share their own stories. Motivational speaker and serial entrepreneur, philosopher and author, in his own words, Dr. Nguyen describes himself as a dentist by circumstances, an entrepreneur by nature and a communicator by passion. He also holds recognitions from the Canadian Parliament and the Canadian Senate.

PAEDIATRIC DENTISTS

From the USA 🇺🇸, **Dr. PAUL DOMINIQUE**, is a paediatric dentist, entrepreneur and investor. He's a graduate of the National University of Ireland, where he earned a Bachelor of Science degree in cell biology and molecular genetics. He completed his dental degree at the University of Kentucky and his specialty training in paediatrics at the Eastman Institute for Oral Health, University of Rochester, NY. Dr. Dominique served as an assistant professor in public health at the University of Kentucky, division of oral health science. During his tenure, he headed and improved a novel mobile program that successfully addresses access to care issues for children in Central and Western Kentucky. Dr. Dominique is also an entrepreneur having acquired and consolidated a small group of practices growing from less than 700K to over 2.4 Million EBITDA in under 24 months. Dr. Dominique has been angel investing for the past decade, investing across a diverse group of platforms such as equity crowdfunding, psychedelic medicine, real estate and teledentistry. He currently serves as a board advisory member to the Teledentists and Revere Partners, the first venture fund dedicated to oral health. He's currently involved in a project that is exploring the use of blockchain technology and NFTs to help improve access to dental care.

From the USA 🇺🇸, **Dr. RICHARD SIMPSON**, DMD, is a board-certified paediatric dentist in private practice and a veteran with 15 years of military service. Dr. Simpson is a Diplomate in the American Board of Paediatric Dentistry, and a Fellow in The American College of Dentists, the International College of Dentists, and the American Academy of Pediatric Dentistry. He has held numerous health professional leadership positions and has experience in state and national cross-sector networking, telehealth/teledentistry, child advocacy, health disparities, policy, and advancing improved medical-dental integration and access to care. He is skilled in leadership, project design and implementation, advocacy, and inter-professional and public-private collaboration. He believes that telehealth is the integral to the future of dentistry and the oral health-overall healthcare paradigm. Dr Simpson is the Immediate Past-Chair of the Oral Health Coalition of Alabama, He serves as and has recently completed his tenure as the Chief Clinical Officer for Holland Healthcare, an international telehealth oral imaging innovator. Dr. Simpson is a member of the Advisory Boards of The TeleDentists and Soluria He and he serves as a Thought Leader and collaborator with TeethCloud, a global oral health initiative dedicated to reducing oral health inequities through technology and DI. Dr. Simpson was recently selected to the 2023 Class of the World's Top 100 Doctors by members of the Global Summits Institute.

From the USA 🇺🇸, **Dr. MARILYN SANDOR**, DDS, MS, is one of Southwest Florida's favourite paediatric dentists. She is highly experienced in her field, having founded her private practice, Naples Paediatric Dentistry in the beautiful community of Naples, Florida in 2001. Dr. Sandor is a successful business owner and an active member of her community. She is committed to educating her young patients on the importance of oral health and enjoys teaching children how to have healthy smiles for a lifetime. Dr. Sandor's paediatric-focused invention, Zooby prophy angles, inspired a full line of creative new products by Young Innovations, which have been bringing joy to dental patients around the world for over a decade. She is the founder and CEO of the GoodCheckup Corporation, a new software company that provides easily accessible and equitable platforms for dentists to expand their reach via a mobile-to-mobile, patent-pending, teledentistry solution. GoodCheckup's flagship products, GoodCheckup Patient and GoodCheckup Doctor are the first Cloud-based, comprehensive smartphone teledentistry applications created by a paediatric dentist specifically for paediatric dentistry.

From the USA 🇺🇸, **Dr. NIDHI TANEJA**, DDS, MSD, is a board-certified paediatric dentist. She is an expert in seeing children with special needs and those with dental fear and anxiety. She wants no child to ever be scared of going to the dentist. Her unique behavior guidance and minimally invasive techniques, help children get through their dental visits with trust and confidence. After being in the conventional model of clinical dentistry which is heavily driven by procedures and surgical intervention, her goal is to help families and children experience dentistry without drills and fears. As a positive childhood advocate, she incorporates mindfulness-based principles in her practice for optimal oral and mental hygiene. She has been awarded 40 under 40 America's Best Dental Specialists, selected for Guiding Leaders program for Women Leadership and is actively involved in organized dentistry with theAmerican Dental Association and the American Academy of Paediatric Dentistry.

From GERMANY 🇩🇪, **Dr. AURORA ALVA**, DMD, is an American board-certified pediatric dentist, a member of the American College of Paediatric Dentists, and a diplomate of the American Board of Paediatric Dentists. She started her career by obtaining a Biology degree from Wellesley College in Wellesley, Massachusetts, where she graduated Cum Laude. During her time at Wellesley, she also had the opportunity to successfully complete courses at the Massachusetts Institute of Technology (MIT) and immersed herself in summer research projects at Harvard Medical School. She obtained various college stipends for her achievements such as from the Howard Hughes Medical Institute, and upon graduation, was one of the two recipients of the Wellesley College Graduate Fellowship Award. She obtained her dental degree and Paediatric Dentistry certificate from Tufts School of Dental Medicine in Boston, Massachusetts, in 2007 and 2009 respectively. Dr. Alva's pediatric dental professional career has been diverse. She has worked in private practice in Massachusetts, Texas and Georgia, participated in humanitarian dental missions in Honduras and Ecuador, worked as a pediatric dental contractor for the American Army in Germany, and worked in private practices in Munich, Germany. Dr. Aurora Alva holds professional licenses from the states of Georgia, Texas, Hawaii, California, Massachustetts and the region of Bavaria in Germany. She is an active member of the American Dental Association, the American Academy of Paediatric Dentists, and the American Board of Pediatric Dentists.

From EGYPT 🇪🇬, **Dr. NOUR AMMAR**, BDS, MS. She is a dedicated specialist in pediatric dentistry and dental public health hailing from Egypt. With an impressive educational background from Alexandria University's Faculty of Dentistry, including graduating top of her class in her bachelor's degree and master's degree, Dr. Ammar has already achieved so much in her field. She has served as a teaching assistant at the same institution for five years, demonstrating her passion for sharing knowledge with others. In addition to her academic accomplishments, Dr. Ammar is also a Harvard alumnus and has participated in a clinical research program there. Her clinical work has earned her several distinguished awards, demonstrating her exceptional skills and commitment to improving patient outcomes. Currently pursuing a Ph.D. at the University of Munich in Germany, Dr. Ammar is committed to raising awareness and knowledge of oral health, particularly among parents and children. Her vision of improving access to dental care for underprivileged or remote populations is being realized through the development of an AI program that can assist primary healthcare centers in identifying different dental pathologies without the real-time presence of a specialist. With her passion for pediatric dentistry and dental public health, Dr. Nour Ammar is a true asset to her profession.

From PERU ▮▮, **Dr. AILIN CABRERA-MATTA**, DDS, MSc, Ph.D., is an associate professor at the Peruvian University Cayetano Heredia. In addition to being a pediatrician, she holds a master's degree in epidemiology, a master's degree in pediatric dentistry, and a doctorate in public health. Her primary interests lie in maternal and child health and the prevention of early childhood caries. She is focused on global health and public health, specifically in relation to children's oral health.

From ITALY ▮ ▮, **Dr. PIERLUIGI PELAGALLI**, DDS, obtained his degree in Dentistry and Dental Prosthetics from the University of Naples Federico II in 1990. He further specialized in Paediatric Dentistry at the University of L'Aquila and focused his training on periodontology, implantology, and prosthetics. Over the years, he has developed a keen interest in paediatric dentistry and new technologies. Dr. Paelagalli received his periodontal surgery and guided tissue regeneration specialization in 1992 from the Royal Dental School in Aarhus, directed by Professor T. Karring. He attended continuing dental education at New York University and various other specialization courses in Oral Surgery and Fixed Prosthesis. He is a student of Dr. Roberto Olivi for children's dentistry. Dr. Paelagalli has been a professor since 2017 at the Master "Fixed prosthesis on natural teeth and implants" at the University of Rome "La Sapienza." He founded the network "the children's dentist" in 2007, and he is interested in promoting the health of children's mouths. Dr. Pelagalli has published several works, including the classification of implant sites and related therapeutic indications, the advantages of using an Er:YAG laser in pedodontics surgery, Kids Cario Test, and Kids Digital Crown Technique. He is a member of various dental societies and is currently working as a freelancer in Rome.

From UNITED ARAB EMIRATES ▭, **Dr. PRRIYA PORWAL**, BDS, MSD, is a paediatric dentist practicing in Abu Dhabi since 2019. She has developed an interest in psychology and clinical hypnotherapy, which she applies to help manage anxiety and uncooperative behaviour of her patients. She has been awarded the Indian Health Professional Awards 2020 for Excellence in Pedodontics. She has been privileged to work with the team of Oncology department in Burjeel Medical City, Abu Dhabi, UAE; as a Specialist Pediatric Dentist, doing Full Mouth Rehabilitation for children requiring Bone Marrow Transplant. . Additionally, she has a strong passion for art, which plays a significant role in her life and influences her approach to dentistry.

PAEDIATRIC DENTISTRY FAQ
ALPHA DENTISTRY vol. 3
ASSEMBLED EDITION

by Dr. BAK NGUYEN, Dr. PAUL DOMINIQUE, Dr. ALVA AURORA
Dr. RICHARD SIMPSON, Dr. MARILYN SANDOR, Dr. NIDHI TANEJA,
Dr. NOUR AMMAR, Dr. AILÍN CABRERA-MATTA, Dr. PRRIYA PORWAL,
and Dr. PIERLUIGI PELAGALLI,

INTRODUCTION
BY Dr. BAK NGUYEN

CONCLUSION
BY Dr. BAK NGUYEN

GLOSSARY OF Dr. BAK's LIBRARY
ANNEX - Dr. BAK NGUYEN

INTRODUCTION

by Dr. BAK NGUYEN

It has been days since the international release of **ALPHA DENTISTRY volume 2**. I am still waiting for the proof of print of my international version to be delivered before sending it to my co-authors from all around the world, their copy. On that, I have great and funny news to share with you.

Let's start with the great news. Well, as of this morning, we are 48 KOLs strong, (key opinion leaders) including myself. If in the first volume, we were 10 international co-authors, we were 11 in the 2nd volume. Well, the bar has been raised for the next one to 12 international authors. The teams are building up and the recruitment of each team is done solely from invitations.

I stand humbled by such international trust and friendships. Within this team alone, Dr. Paul Dominique, Dr. Aurora Alva, Dr. Richard Simpson and Dr. Marilyn Sandor all went above and beyond to recruit international experts and Alphas. My friends, you have my deepest gratitude.

Another great news is that we have also raised the bar of speed and production. If the first volume took 11 months to complete, thanks to the advancement in technology and Artificial Intelligence, volume 2 took 2 months and a half, from the first interview to the book being distributed internationally in 51 countries, in electronic and printed forms. Yes, you can go online and search for **ALPHA DENTISTRY vol. 2 - IMPLANTOLOGY FAQ** and can have your own copy delivered to your doors.

That said, I am upholding my promise, a PDF copy will be made available shortly for everyone to download, free of charge. Those were part of the rules of engagement of this project. Well, that promise and the chance to contribute to the world's first crowdsourcing dental knowledge base echoed around the planet and found its appeal. Within the last 2 weeks, as the co-authors of team ALPHA 2 were celebrating the release of their volume, we nearly doubled in KOLs numbers, recruiting for the next 6 teams.

This is proof that speed is really one of my powers. Going that fast, we kept friction and resistance at a minimum while building up international momentum and appeal. That also changed the course within team ALPHA 2 itself.

"Action inspires even more actions"
Dr. Bak Nguyen

Responding to the growing momentum, members of ALPHA 2, led by Dr. Gurien Demiraqi, started taking more and more versions upon their shoulders. Dr. Demiraqi opened the race by volunteering to cover 2 other tongues (German and Italian) on top of English and Albanian. Then, Dr. Bennete Fernandes proposed to take 4 too.

What started as a reach in the first volume, as I was looking to be useful to dentists outside of America, today has become an inherited landmark signature of the ALPHAS. During our celebrations on an international Podcast, it was really well underlined how including other tongues increased exponentially the appeal of this collaborative work, making it even more inclusive.

Well, that came with its toll of workload. I was okay with that. The final version compiled 11 KOLs, 247 years of experience, more than 240K words, authors from 8 different countries, and partially translated into 11 different tongues! That's impressive, very impressive when you think that in my first year as an author, I wrote less than 250K words combined! And here's a funny anecdote!

The compiled version, called the INTERNATIONAL version, was 940+ pages thick. Well, at submission, I learnt that the maximum number of pages that Amazon allows was 828 pages! We were more than 100 pages over the maximum allowed by Amazon! It took 4 revisions and 6 hours to trim 140 pages from the final version. It was painful, but we successfully got it right without cutting any content out!

So today, I gain a new story to tell: we broke Amazon's ceiling! Isn't that a testimony to the force of our collective minds, to what it means to be ALPHAS?

It is with that motivation that I am back in mission control with the international crew of ALPHA 3: the paediatric volume. Please join me to welcoming: returning co-authors, from the USA, Dr. Paul Dominique and from the Germany, Dr. Aurora Alva; from the USA, Dr. Richard Simpson, Dr. Marilyn Sandor, and Dr. Nidhi Taneja; from Egypt, Dr. Nour Ammar; from Italy, Pierluigi Pelagalli, from Peru, Dr. Ailin Cabrera-Matta, and from the United Arab Emirates, Dr. Prriya Porwal.

You see, I did not wait for the last mission to be completed before launching this one. While I was waiting for the revision of the members of ALPHA 2, I started the interview process for ALPHA 3. Yes, even if we leveraged artificial intelligence, we have to write each of the words contained in these books, more than once! So no, AI did not write the book for us. We just worked smarter.

Going through the interview process, I noticed how kind each paediatric doctor was. I am not polite here; really, the way they approached the answers was profoundly different than the other team, much more human, dipped in tenderness! This goes well beyond the personality of each, it is rooted in their training and core.

Here's what I meant by that. If the kindness was general and standardized, there was a question where they were asked why adults should not share utensils or drinks with their child. All of the doctors of ALPHA 2 find ways to explain in length the reasons. Well, I could see the effort they all put in to avoid saying what all the other doctors would have answered with a single word, myself included: contamination!

For now 5 years, I was researching for ways to rebuild our profession. Especially after COVID, I was actively seeking ways to fix our public image. Well, working with so many dentists, I can state with confidence that if we come together as a profession, the spoke people should be amongst the paediatric dentists!

That understanding inspired me to explore new possibilities. I got creative and gave in to it. I leveraged my skills as a producer and borrowed from my artistic side and the advancement in artificial intelligence to theme this book in PIXAR-DISNEY's style. I even got 3D avatars made, inspired by each of the members of ALPHA 2. They all adored the bold initiative!

Just like the other volumes, each co-author will be answering the same patients' FAQ (Frequently Asked Questions) and will be doing so just as if they were talking to the patients themselves, or, in this case, to their parents.

This information has been conceived and gathered keeping the perspective of the patients at its focus, making the wording and explanation as easy to understand as possible. In my lexicon, I call that humanizing our science and knowledge.

It is my joy and privilege to present to you the 3rd volume of **ALPHA DENTISTRY** and its international cast: Dr.

Dominique, Dr. Alva, Dr. Simpson, Dr. Sandor, Dr. Taneja, Dr. Ammar, Dr. Pelagalli

Dr. Cabrera-Matta, Dr. Porwal, thank you for your dedication.

This is **ALPHA DENTISTRY vol. 3, PAEDIATRIC DENTISTRY FAQ**. Welcome to the Alphas.

Dr. BAK NGUYEN

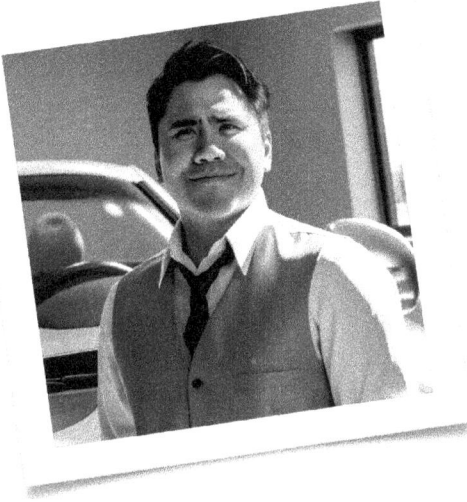

Dr. BAK NGUYEN,
DMD

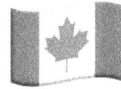

From Canada, **Dr. BAK NGUYEN,** Nominee Ernst and Young Entrepreneur of the year, Grand Homage Lys DIVERSITY, LinkedIn & TownHall Achiever of the year and TOP 100 Doctors 2021. In 2023, he made the CREA GLOBAL AWARD list. Dr. Bak is a cosmetic dentist, CEO and founder of Mdex & Co. His company is revolutionizing the dental field. Speaker and motivator, he holds the world record of writing 120 books in 5 years accumulating many world records (to be officialized). Before that, he held the world record of writing 9 books over 12 months, then, 15 books within 15 months to set the bar even higher with the world record of 36 books written within 18 months + 1 week. By his second author anniversary, he scored his new landmark world record of 48 books within 24 months. And then 72 books in 36 months. By the 4th anniversary, Dr. Bak scored his usual landmark of writing 96 books over 48 months, but he pushed even further, scoring also the landmark world record of 100 books written within 4 years and then, 120 books written in 5 years! In 2003, he founded Mdex, a dental company upon which in 2018, he launched the most ambitious private endeavour to reform the dental industry, Canada-wide. Philosopher, he has close to his heart the quest of happiness of the people surrounding him, patients and colleagues alike. In 2020, he launched an International collaborative initiative named **THE ALPHAS** to share knowledge and for Entrepreneurs and Doctors to thrive through the Greatest Pandemic and Economic depression of our time.

In 2016, he co-found with Tranie Vo, Emotive World Incorporated, a tech research company to use technology to empower happiness and sharing. U.A.X. the ultimate audio experience is the landmark project on which the team is advancing, utilizing the technics of the movie industry and the advancement in ARTIFICIAL INTELLIGENCE to save the book industry and upgrade the continuing education space. These projects have allowed Dr. Nguyen to attract interest from the international and diplomatic community and he is now the centre of a global discussion on the wellbeing and the future of the health profession. It is in that matter that he shares his thoughts and encourages the health community to share their own stories. Motivational speaker and serial entrepreneur, philosopher and author, in his own words, Dr. Nguyen describes himself as a dentist by circumstances, an entrepreneur by nature and a communicator by passion. He also holds recognitions from the Canadian Parliament and the Canadian Senate.

Dr. Bak Nguyen is a prolific dentist, entrepreneur and an epic character. He is the CEO of Mdex in Montreal, Canada and has a litany of accolades, including CREA Global Award, World Top100 Doctor, EY Nominee for Entrepreneur of the year, Grand Homage LYS DIVERSITY, and LinkedIn & TownHall Achiever of the year. Dr. Nguyen is also an enthusiastic author, holding the World Record for publishing 100 books in 4 years.

I had the great fortune to meet Bak during the COVID lockdowns. After our initial conversations, it was very clear to me that Bak was poised to become a global leader, inspiring a new generation of dentists in the post-pandemic era and more importantly, we would become lifelong friends.

Bak clearly perceives that accessibility is one of the major hurdles facing the dental profession on a global scale. He is empathetic to suffering, being aware that children are a vulnerable population and that a new era of advocacy is sorely needed. He realizes that a new paradigm is needed in paediatric dentistry.

To that effect, he is helping to drive the narrative toward a new, technologically advanced and preventive approach that will eventually make the current system irrelevant and redundant. I am always honoured and privileged to collaborate with my great colleague from up north.

Dr. Paul Dominique

This is **ALPHA DENTISTRY vol. 3, PAEDIATRIC DENTISTRY FAQ**. Welcome to the Alphas.

Dr. BAK NGUYEN

CHAPTER 1

"PAEDIATRIC DENTISTRY"

by Dr. BAK NGUYEN

FROM CANADA

DISCLOSURE: Since PAEDIATRIC is not my field of expertise, I am writing all of the following answers after the interviews and reviews of my colleagues. I am also including all of their answers in mine to cover as much fields as possible.

1.1 - DEFINITIONS

by Dr. BAK NGUYEN FROM CANADA 🇨🇦

WHAT IS THE BEST TYPE OF TOOTHBRUSH FOR MY CHILD?
I will say the toothbrush that they will be using. Just like with adults, a soft toothbrush is always recommended and one they will take an interest in using. If for adults, a toothbrush is a tool, for a child, it can be a symbol. To miss that would be a huge oversight. As for electronic toothbrushes, I will say the same too, for both adults and kids. If that kind of upgrade can motivate you to take better care of your teeth, by all means!

WHAT IS THE ROLE OF FLUORIDE IN PREVENTING CAVITIES?
Fluoride strengthens teeth by making them resistant to acid attacks from bacteria in plaque, preventing cavities. It can reverse early stages of tooth decay by remineralizing enamel. Fluoride can be obtained through various sources such as drinking water, toothpaste, mouthwash, and professional treatments. It is added to public water supplies in many areas. Professional fluoride treatments are recommended for those at high risk for cavities. Regular use of fluoride is an effective way to maintain good oral health.

WHAT IS THE DIFFERENCE BETWEEN A PAEDIATRIC DENTIST AND A GENERAL DENTIST?
A paediatric dentist is a dentist specialized in children's cares. Much more than about treating children's teeth and illness, they have a special interest in

communicating with the children and their parents. That is a unique set of skills that paediatric dentists master. Other than that, they are treating children on a daily basis, so their have access to the right equipment, expertise, and supporting staff.

WHAT ARE THE MOST COMMON ORTHODONTIC PROBLEMS IN CHILDREN?

To a parent, the most common orthodontic problem is teeth alignment, especially as children are transiting from their primary teeth into their permanent teeth. That is often not a problem, since growth will catch up and fix most of the present issues. So yes, all children go through a phase where their teeth do not look that great. That said, it is not a universal truth. Some children will present bone discrepancy and growth issues. These are to be diagnosed as soon as possible and to be addressed while the child's growth can still be leveraged in our favour. So in a simple answer, the most common orthodontic problem in a child is often not what the parents think. The bone and growth issues are usually identified by the attending paediatric dentist or dentist. This is why it is important to have regular following-up with your attending.

HOW CAN I TELL IF MY CHILD NEEDS ORTHODONTIC TREATMENT?

In children's orthodontic, the obvious is not always the truth. When a young child (2-5 year-old) has a perfect smile, that is usually not a problem to their parents while in fact, that child might have a severe tendency to misalignment as soon as the permanent teeth are arriving. That *early perfect smile* was misleading. In the same line of thought, when a child presents misalignment and even 2 rows of teeth while in transition between the eruption of their permanent teeth, is not something to be alarmed with. This happens because the growth of the face and jaws aren't completed yet as the permanent teeth coming out have their permanent size. So again, it can be very misleading. The answer to this question is to have your children monitored by their attending paediatric dentists or dentists, they will tell you if something is an issue.

WHAT ARE THE BENEFITS OF DENTAL SEALANTS FOR CHILDREN?

A dental sealant is an artificial mechanical coat of protection for the occlusal face (the surface used to masticate) of the posterior teeth. The wide use of sealants is not universal as some dentists and paediatric dentists will recommend them only is certain situations while other doctors will use them as a universal layer for prevention. As a parent, what is important to understand, is that dental sealants are a layer of protection, not a warranty, problem-free solution.

Sealants is technique sensitive and demand the proper experience and technique. That said, dental sealants are wearing down as the child is chewing, just like winter tires, they are not forever! As of for the cost of dental sealants, they are cheaper than a restoration but they still cost money. If you ask me, money for prevention is always a good investment, not it will be for you to make that decision. Prevention, not warranty!

1.2 - PREVENTION

by Dr. BAK NGUYEN FROM CANADA 🇨🇦

HOW CAN I PREPARE MY CHILD FOR THEIR FIRST DENTAL VISIT?

The best approach is not to make a big deal out of the visit. Often, the child will mimic the perspective of their parents. So if it is not a big deal, the child will go through the experience without bias and will have the chance to make his or her own opinion about dentistry. If the parent was fearful, that fear will be picked up by the child and that will make their own dental experience must harder. The stratagem to not make a big deal out of it, either before or after is a winning strategy. I will take this opportunity to emphasize that if you wait for a problem to occur, an infection to solve, that first contact with the dentist will not be the best of experience. Therefore, prevention is key!

HOW CAN I HELP MY CHILD OVERCOME THEIR FEAR OF THE DENTIST?

Your child is not born with the fear of the dentist. That fear has either been transferred by you or those close to the child or happened because you waited for an emergency to happen, one requiring a surgical intervention. As you can imagine, that first contact will be etched into the child's mind as a trauma. Consult paediatric dentists and dentists for prevention and don't make a big deal out of these visits are the key to not traumatize your child.

IS IT OKAY FOR CHILDREN TO CONSUME SUGARY FOODS AND DRINKS?

We are who we are. It would be nearly impossible to avoid all sugary foods and drinks. My advice is to be aware that those will cause harm to your child if not monitored and care for (dental hygiene) after consumption. The rule should be that after every sugary intake, they or you, should clean their teeth. That said, it will not be feasible to brush the teeth at that frequency, so try to manage the frequency of sugary intake to a manageable habit. SUGAR, then, BRUSHING! That's the equation.

HOW CAN I ENSURE MY CHILD IS GETTING ENOUGH FLUORIDE?

In North America, fluoride has been incorporated into so many of our daily product. Even if the water of your municipality is not added with fluoride, just brushing the teeth with the popular brand of toothpaste is usually enough for your child. Unless a personalized diagnosis by the attending paediatric dentist or physician tells you otherwise, you do not have to worry. Consult your attending and follow their instructions.

CAN MY CHILD STILL ENJOY SWEET TREATS WHILE MAINTAINING GOOD ORAL HYGIENE?

It would be nearly impossible to avoid all sugary foods and drinks. My advice is to be aware that those will cause harm to your child if not monitored and care for (dental hygiene) after consumption. The rule should be that after every sugary intake, they or you, should clean their teeth. That said, it will not be feasible to brush the teeth at that frequency, so try to manage the frequency of sugary intake to a manageable habit. SUGAR, then, BRUSHING! That's the equation.

HOW CAN I PREVENT ORTHODONTIC PROBLEMS IN MY CHILD?

Orthodontic problems have 2 origins: genes and habits. The gene's part is not addressable, they will present the combination of their parents' genes. Those will need to be addressed at the proper timing. Once again, monitoring is key. In the case of habits, those can be addressed. The most damaging habit is thumb-sucking or the overuse of pacifiers. If those were acceptable to all children, from the age of 2 and above, as soon as possible, parents should take the initiative to stop these habits. Thumb-sucking, for example, is the continued application of a force forward on the upper palette and the upper front teeth while applying a lower pressure on the lower jaw and the anterior teeth. These will affect the development of the child's jaws.

HOW CAN I PREPARE MY CHILD FOR A DENTAL PROCEDURE?

Just like any visit to the dentist, you should not make a big deal of going to the dentist, neither before nor after. Let the child makes his or her own impression. Most paediatric dentists are particularly trained to make the experience as smooth as possible, so just let it be.

HOW CAN I ENSURE MY CHILD IS RECEIVING ADEQUATE NUTRITION FOR HEALTHY TEETH?

It is important to give your child a balanced diet with a variety of foods from all food groups, including calcium, vitamin D, and phosphorus-rich foods. Limiting sugary and acidic foods and drinks can help prevent tooth decay. Drinking water and brushing teeth with fluoride toothpaste twice a day are also recommended. Regular dental check-ups can help monitor oral health and nutrition for healthy teeth.

by Dr. BAK NGUYEN FROM CANADA 🇨🇦

WHAT IS THE BEST AGE FOR A CHILD TO START SEEING A DENTIST?
Paediatric dentists like to see the child as soon as possible. The first tooth eruption is often the rallying call. Remember that the goal of a paediatric dentist goes way beyond treating teeth, it is about easing the parents and the child into the proper way to handle their dental health. And how important is the dental health of a child? Well, the mouth is the entry point of food, by extension growth and all the pleasure of eating. If that is not enough to convince you, the mouth is also the entry point to your body, with its microbial flora. Ti take care of the dental health of your child is to save them from worlds of potential troubles, for them and for you!

HOW OFTEN SHOULD MY CHILD SEE A DENTIST?
Once the primary contact made, the attending dentist will tell you at what frequency you should have your child in, based on the specific needs of your child. A general rule would be every 6 months if nothing is outside of the norms.

WHAT IS THE BEST AGE FOR A CHILD TO GET ORTHODONTIC TREATMENT?
This is a tricky question. It depends on the problem of that child. The only general rules here would be to break the damaging habits (thumb-sucking and overuse of pacifiers) as soon as possible from age 2 and

above, to maintain a healthy mouth preventing the premature loss of baby teeth, and to address bone discrepancy issues before puberty. Again, these can only be diagnosed and addressed by your attending.

WHAT ARE THE SIGNS OF TEETH ERUPTION IN A CHILD?
As a child's teeth begin to emerge, you may notice some signs such as excessive drooling, fussiness, swollen or red gums, and the tendency to bite or chew on objects. Additionally, a small white bump or tooth may appear through the gums. Some children may also experience mild fever or diarrhea during this process. However, it's important to keep in mind that every child is unique and may exhibit varied symptoms during teeth eruption.

1.4 - MAINTENANCE

by Dr. BAK NGUYEN FROM CANADA 🍁

WHAT IS THE RIGHT WAY TO CLEAN MY CHILD'S TEETH?
To clean your child's teeth properly, you should use a soft-bristled toothbrush and a little bit of fluoride toothpaste. For children under three years old, apply a smear of toothpaste that is the size of a grain of rice. For children aged three to six, use a pea-sized amount of toothpaste. Brush their teeth twice a day in a circular motion, ensuring that you clean all surfaces of the teeth and gums. Encourage your child to spit out the toothpaste after brushing, but do not let them rinse

their mouth with water. Flossing should be done once a day for children with two teeth that touch. Regular dental check-ups with a paediatric dentist can also help maintain proper dental hygiene and identify any potential issues early on.

HOW CAN I ENCOURAGE MY CHILD TO BRUSH THEIR TEETH REGULARLY?
Monkey sees, monkey do! That should be the theme. Have them to join you as you are burning your own teeth. If there are too young, brush their teeth but have them see you brush yours too! If this is a regular activity, even a bonding opportunity, it will grow into the life habit that everyone should have to spare yourself and them from dental pain. As a parent, address everything with positivity, fear is not the best approach here.

HOW CAN I PREVENT TOOTH DECAY IN MY CHILD'S BABY TEETH?
The baby teeth are much thinner as far as the enamel goes. Good hygiene and the management of sugary intakes are the steps in the good direction. That said, try to avoid as much as possible sugary drinks, especially in the bottle. These will be catastrophic in the long run on your children teeth.

HOW CAN I PREVENT MY CHILD FROM DEVELOPING DENTAL ANXIETY?
Of course, by not making a big deal of the dental visit. Do not address teeth nor dental care from fear, and above all, do not transfer your own fear of the dentist!

HOW CAN I HELP MY CHILD AVOID DENTAL INJURIES?
Children move, run and fall. That is a part of life. Sure, as parents, we all want to keep them safe, but they will all

learn from their own mistakes, that is part of building their confidence. One single advise on the matter is to have your child not showing their teeth while swimming, running, even walking fast. If they are old enough to practice contact sports, have mouthguards made.

HOW CAN I HELP MY CHILD AVOID GUM DISEASE?

Gum disease occurs and the food accumulates between the teeth and the gum. Well, most children will present spaces in between their teeth until the arrival of the permanent teeth. These spaces prevent the accumulation of food, so just by brushing the teeth, the adequate hygiene will be obtained. Dental floss should be used as soon as the teeth come in contact. Flossing will dislodge the food track between the teeth.

HOW CAN I HELP MY CHILD MAINTAIN GOOD ORAL HYGIENE WHILE WEARING BRACES?

While wearing braces and orthodontic appliances, the hygiene is key, not just on the teeth, but the gums and the appliances too. It is always about keeping the surface clean of biofilm and food residues. As your kid will receive their braces or appliances, the orthodontists and their staff will instruct them on how to keep proper hygiene.

HOW CAN I HELP MY CHILD AVOID TOOTH SENSITIVITY?

Sure, most sensitivities in a child are caries related, except for teeth eruption and injuries. To keep good hygiene, to avoid sugary drinks, especially in the bottle, and to have your children regularly followed by their attending are the steps to prevent teeth problems, therefore sensitivity in a broad sense.

1.5 - DENTAL WORK

by Dr. BAK NGUYEN FROM CANADA 🍁

WHAT ARE THE MOST COMMON DENTAL PROBLEMS IN CHILDREN?

Dental caries is the most common and trending problem in children. The problem with teeth is that it does not hurt until it is too late. The reason why prevention is so important in paediatric cares is that since all the teeth in the mouth are receiving the same treatment, problems never come alone. And if we wait for pain as a call to action, it is often extensive treatments. So much can be avoid with so little…

WHAT CAN I DO IF MY CHILD HAS A DENTAL EMERGENCY?

The best place to think of as a child presents a dental emergency is the dental clinic in which he or she is followed. Paediatric dentists call those, dental homes. That would be the best option. Having access to a regular dentist is also an excellent option. Nowadays, there are also tele-dentistry services that can be very useful, especially to have quick answers. Most hospital emergencies do not have dental services or dental staff, so dental-wise, it is not the best of options.

IS IT NECESSARY FOR MY CHILD TO HAVE DENTAL X-RAYS TAKEN?

X-rays allow attending to see the bones and through the different layers of the teeth. Without x-rays, it is very hard to assess the condition of the bone, the development of the teeth to erupt nor the cavities starting. Especially with digital x-rays, the emitted doses

39

are minimal and safe under the care of attending doctors. And yes, x-rays are part of the essentials for monitoring the dental health of your child.

WHAT IS THE BEST WAY TO TREAT A CHILD'S CAVITIES?
The first thing with a cavity is to stop the active process. Cleaning the cavity and removing the infected part is the first step. If the cavity was affecting only the superior layers of the tooth (enamel and dentine), a filling will be used to restore the tooth. There are different filling materials possible (glass ionomer, composite, amalgame). Each has its indication. The choice of therapy will fall on the attending to choose the best course of action.

If the damage are more extensive but the teeth are still salvageable, the use of metal crowns becomes the alternative most paediatric dentists will suggest. Those are metal crowns that will protect the teeth while restoring their function until the replacement of these teeth with their permanent counterparts. In the case that the cavity is too extensive, extraction might be the only solution of treatment. When that is the case, space maintainers therapy will be necessary to prevent future orthodontic problems.

WHAT IS DENTAL SEALANT, AND IS IT NECESSARY FOR MY CHILD?
A dental sealant is an artificial mechanical coat of protection for the occlusal face (the surface used to masticate) of the posterior teeth. The wide use of sealants is not universal as some dentists and paediatric dentists will recommend them only is certain situations while other doctors will use them as a universal layer for prevention. As a parent, what is important to

understand, is that dental sealants are a layer of protection, not a warranty, problem-free solution. Sealants is technique sensitive and demand the proper experience and technique. That said, dental sealants are wearing down as the child is chewing, just like winter tires, they are not forever! As of for the cost of dental sealants, they are cheaper than a restoration but they still cost money. If you ask me, money for prevention is always a good investment, not it will be for you to make that decision. Prevention, not warranty!

WHAT ARE THE BENEFITS OF ORTHODONTIC TREATMENT FOR CHILDREN?
Orthodontic treatment can provide many benefits for children. The most significant advantage is the improvement of teeth and jaw alignment, which can enhance the appearance and function of the mouth. Straighter teeth are easier to clean, reducing the risk of tooth decay and gum disease. Correcting orthodontic issues early on can also improve a child's bite, preventing speech, eating, and jaw pain problems. This early intervention can prevent more severe problems from developing in the future and potentially reduce the need for extensive and costly treatment later on. Finally, having a healthier, straighter smile can boost a child's self-esteem and confidence, leading to better social interactions and an overall improvement in their quality of life.

IS IT OKAY FOR MY CHILD TO PLAY SPORTS WITH BRACES?
Of course, we just need to take the necessary precaution to prevent and injuries. Mouthguards are usually the protection needed. In the case that a child is having a headgear (an orthodontic appliance with external component), well, it would be advised for the

child not to wear his or her headgear will practicing that sport. The mouthguard only protect the teeth inside of the mouth, not the external appliance. The general rule will be that anything not fixed in the mouth should be removed while practicing sport.

WHAT ARE THE RISKS OF NOT TREATING MY CHILD'S CAVITIES?

The obvious risk of not treating a cavity is the worsening of that cavity which can lead to pain, infection, and the loss of that tooth. Big deal, may you say. Well, in simple cases, that premature loss will affect the growth of the jaw and cause orthodontic issues to be addressed later on. That will be expensive and easily avoided.

In extreme cases, the infection resulting from the dental cavity could spread in the bloodstream and be responsible for much extensive health damage. There are cases that lead to the death of the patient (child). It is on that premise that North American governments have included child dental care to a certain extent. That was in the effort to avoid fatal complications while the starting point was so easy to fix.

HOW CAN I PREVENT BABY BOTTLE TOOTH DECAY IN MY CHILD?

Well, to prevent baby bottle tooth decay, just give nothing but water in the bottle of that child. Sure, milk, breast milk, and formula milk are usually what is contained in these bottles. Well, you should have the child to feed, then clean their teeth before letting go to sleep. As soon as the teeth have erupted, even milk could natural sugar that will cause tooth decay.

The worse situations are parents who leave their kids with juice in the bottle that the child can have all and long. Even worse, to have them sleep with juice bottles to fall asleep. No child should be drinking into sleep, not even milk! Preventing that should keep your child from developing baby bottle decay.

HOW CAN I FIND A PAEDIATRIC DENTIST FOR MY CHILD?

The most common way will be a web research on the internet. Paediatric Dentists can also be found on the website of the official dental organization of the state or of the province. If you have a dentist, you can also be referred by your dentist to a paediatric dentist.

HOW CAN I HELP MY CHILD MAINTAIN GOOD ORAL HYGIENE WHILE WEARING APPLIANCES?

While wearing braces and orthodontic appliances, the hygiene is key, not just on the teeth, but the gums and the appliances too. It is always about keeping the surface clean of biofilm and food residues. As your kid will receive their braces or appliances, the orthodontists and their staff will instruct them on how to keep proper hygiene.

1.6 - FEAR/PAIN

by Dr. BAK NGUYEN FROM CANADA 🇨🇦

IS SEDATION DENTISTRY NECESSARY FOR CHILDREN?

The need for sedation dentistry in children varies based on factors such as their age, anxiety levels, and the dental procedure they require. Sedation may be necessary for kids who are fearful or anxious about dental procedures, have trouble sitting still, or need extensive dental work. However, it's crucial to use sedation only when necessary and with caution, considering the potential risks. A qualified dentist or paediatric dentist should evaluate the child's individual needs and medical history to decide whether to use sedation.

HOW CAN I HELP MY CHILD COPE WITH TOOTH LOSS?

When children lose their teeth, it's important to comfort them and let them know it's a normal part of growing up. Encourage them to talk to you about any worries they may have and make a special tradition for the Tooth Fairy to celebrate each lost tooth. You can also provide cold washcloths or teething toys to ease any discomfort and emphasize the importance of good oral hygiene and nutrition. If necessary, don't hesitate to seek advice from a paediatric dentist or therapist for additional support.

HOW CAN I RELIEVE MY CHILD'S TOOTH ERUPTION PAIN?

If your child is experiencing tooth eruption pain, there are some methods that can help alleviate their discomfort. Offering a cold towel, teething toy, or chilled spoon can provide temporary relief. If your child is still uncomfortable, over-the-counter pain medication may be given. However, it is crucial to avoid using any teething gels or creams as they may not offer any additional benefits and could potentially harm your child.

WHAT ARE THE RISKS OF USING TEETHING GELS AND CREAMS?

It is important to be aware of the potential risks associated with using teething gels and creams. These products may contain benzocaine, which can lead to a serious condition known as methemoglobinemia, particularly in children under two years of age. Additionally, teething gels and creams can cause irritation to the gums and may worsen the teething pain. As a result, pediatric dentists typically advise against the use of these products and recommend alternative methods for soothing teething discomfort.

HOW CAN I HELP MY CHILD RECOVER AFTER A DENTAL PROCEDURE?

The most important part after dental treatment is the numbness period that follows dental surgery. Well, make sure that your child does not bite him or herself. Since they are numb, they might bite their chick or lips. After a few hours, the effect of the local anesthetic will fade and your child is now back to normal. In the case of amalgam despair, your child will have to chew on the other side for 24 hours. You will have to remind him or her about that too. In simple terms, following the post-op instruction of your dentist should keep the recovering process smooth.

1.7 - MONEY

by Dr. BAK NGUYEN FROM CANADA 🇨🇦

WHAT IS THE COST OF PAEDIATRIC DENTAL CARE?

It is a false belief to think that paediatric cares are less expensive than adult cares. Of course, the cares are not exactly the same, it is difficult to compare, but a filling of a child is pretty comparable to the filling of an adult. If anything, it might require more procedures like sedation or special techniques that will be added to the fees. One sure thing, prevention is much less costly. In that instance, dental sealants are cheaper than fillings and metal crowns!

ARE THOSE COVERED BY THE GOVERNMENT?
In North America, most provinces or states have coverage that will cover children's dental care up to a certain extent. The specification and the coverage are to be verified with your state or provincial authorities.

ARE INSURANCE COVERING CHILD DENTAL CARE?
Usually, private insurance will cover what is not covered by the state or provincial children's benefits program. That said, it is for you to verify with your insurance company what is covered and what is not covered. Private insurances have their specific terms and programs. You will have to enquire about your specific benefits.

1.8 - HABITS

by Dr. BAK NGUYEN FROM CANADA 🇨🇦

IS THUMB-SUCKING HARMFUL TO MY CHILD'S TEETH?

Absolutely. Thumb-sucking is the number habit that will cause your child to have orthodontic issues. Passed the age of 2, you should stop your child from sucking his or her thumb or keep using pacifiers.

HOW CAN I ENCOURAGE MY CHILD TO STOP THUMB-SUCKING?

The easiest way will be to pull his or her thumb out from age 2 and above. The longer a child will be sucking his or her thumb, the harder it will be to break the habit. When it comes to breaking the habits, there are different methods and different appliances that could help, all of which have to be prescribed by your attending. Pull his or her thumb out as soon as possible after the age of 2 to prevent the formation of a habit and you will be avoid complications.

HOW CAN I PREVENT MY CHILD FROM GRINDING THEIR TEETH AT NIGHT?

Teeth grinding is not a habit that can be addressed, at least not at a child level. If that only happens once, you can rest reassured. If this happens all the time, please see your attending to discuss the cause and how to rectify the problem.

WHAT ARE THE DANGERS OF SHARING UTENSILS AND DRINKS WITH MY CHILD?

Sharing utensils and drink with your child will transfer the bacteria in your mouth down to your child. In that sense, an adult with the prompt to much dental decay will transfer his or her bacteria down to the child, sharing spoons, utensils, and drinks.

HOW CAN I HELP MY CHILD AVOID JAW PROBLEMS?

Jaws problems are often gene-related. Those cannot be prevented. Habits-related issues leading to jaw development problems such as thumb-sucking can, on the other hand, be prevented by stopping the habit a young age, or by breaking the habit before the damage becomes extensive and permanent in the growth of the jaws.

HOW CAN I PREVENT DENTAL PROBLEMS IN MY CHILD WHILE THEY ARE SLEEPING?

As a responsible parent, there are two dental problems that you can prevent while your child is asleep. Firstly, avoid giving them a bottle of milk or juice to drink as they fall asleep. Secondly, it's crucial to break the habit of thumb-sucking before they turn two. If your child continues to suck their thumb during sleep, gently remove their hand and educate them on the importance of avoiding this habit. You can also cover their fingers to discourage thumb-sucking.

This is **ALPHA DENTISTRY vol. 3, PAEDIATRIC DENTISTRY FAQ**. Welcome to the Alphas.

Dr. BAK NGUYEN

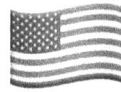

Dr. PAUL DOMINIQUE,
DDS, MS

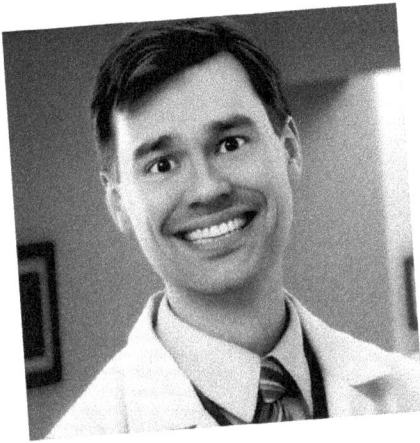

From the USA 🇺🇸, **Dr. PAUL DOMINIQUE**, is a paediatric dentist, entrepreneur and investor. He's a graduate of the National University of Ireland, where he earned a Bachelor of Science degree in cell biology and molecular genetics. He completed his dental degree at the University of Kentucky and his specialty training in paediatrics at the Eastman Institute for Oral Health, University of Rochester, NY. Dr. Dominique served as an assistant professor in public health at the University of Kentucky, division of oral health science. During his tenure, he headed and improved a novel mobile program that successfully addresses access to care issues for children in Central and Western Kentucky. Dr. Dominique is also an entrepreneur having acquired and consolidated a small group of practices growing from less than 700K to over 2.4 Million EBITDA in under 24 months. Dr. Dominique has been angel investing for the past decade, investing across a diverse group of platforms such as equity crowdfunding, psychedelic medicine, real estate and teledentistry. He currently serves as a board advisory member to the Teledentists and Revere Partners, the first venture fund dedicated to oral health. He's currently involved in a project that is exploring the use of blockchain technology and NFTs to help improve access to dental care.

Paul and I met at the beginning of the COVID pandemic, back when, as dentists, we were all lost and looking for answers. Paul is amongst the first Alpha doctors who joined the Alphas as we started organizing to rebuild our profession.

Needless to say, we became good friends. Visionary and impactful entrepreneur, Dr. Dominique is amongst the smartest people that I have the privilege to exchange and build with. He is insightful, creative, and does not stop for any boundaries. In a conservative profession like ours, we need courageous and out-of-the-box thinkers like Dr. Paul Dominique.

Paul has been a founding member of the Alphas as well as a great recruiter of the co-authors of this series. He is a sharp mind to bounce ideas with, a true friend who always had my back, and a great conversation when it comes to looking for impossible solutions.

I am privileged to serve with Alpha doctors of the calibre of Dr. Paul Dominique. Please join me to welcome Alpha Dr. Paul Dominique.

Dr. Bak Nguyen

This is **ALPHA DENTISTRY vol. 3, PAEDIATRIC DENTISTRY FAQ**.
Welcome to the Alphas.

CHAPTER 2

"PAEDIATRIC DENTISTRY"

by Dr. PAUL DOMINIQUE

FROM USA 🇺🇸

2.1 - DEFINITIONS

by Dr. PAUL DOMINIQUE FROM USA 🇺🇸

WHAT IS THE BEST TYPE OF TOOTHBRUSH FOR MY CHILD?

When selecting a toothbrush for your child, it is best to choose one with a small head and soft bristles. This allows for easy access to the back teeth and reduces the risk of damaging the gums. As for electric toothbrushes, I'm in different to them, I'm neither for them or against them. One can do just a good job with a manual toothbrush, if used judiciously. However, one has to take extra care with a rotary brush head as it can lead to gum recession with improper use.

WHAT IS THE ROLE OF FLUORIDE IN PREVENTING CAVITIES?

Fluoride plays three important roles in preventing cavities. Its mechanism of action is purely topical. Firstly, it promotes remineralization of the enamel, which strengthens the teeth. Secondly, it prevents the demineralization of the enamel, which helps protect the teeth from decay. Lastly, fluoride is bacteriostatic. This helps to prevent the growth of bacteria in the mouth. In summary, fluoride promotes remineralization, prevents demineralization, and is bacteriostatic.

WHAT IS THE DIFFERENCE BETWEEN A PAEDIATRIC DENTIST AND A GENERAL DENTIST?

Paediatric dentistry is and age defined specialty of dentistry and a subspecialty of paediatrics. It is the branch of dentistry that deals with patients from birth through adolescents and also adults with intellectual disabilities or special needs. A paediatric dentist is a specialist dentist who spends two or more years of advanced supervised training at the post doctoral level, after completing a dental degree. This is the primary difference between a paediatric dentist and a general dentist. The specialty training that a paediatric dentist undertakes is traditionally referred to a residency program.

This program provides specialised training in the oral healthcare needs of children, taking into consideration. their unique physiological , emotional, and developmental needs. A paediatric dentist is trained to manage a wide range of dental issues in children, including preventative care, restorative treatments, interceptive & comprehensive orthodontics and dental emergencies. They also have expertise in working with children with special needs or dental anxiety. The goal of a paediatric dentist is to provide comprehensive and individualised care that promotes good oral health and encourages a positive attitude towards dental care in children.

WHAT ARE THE MOST COMMON ORTHODONTIC PROBLEMS IN CHILDREN?

In my experience as a paediatric dentist, the most common orthodontic issues I see in children are related to habits such as thumb sucking and tongue thrusting or protrusion. These habits can cause misalignment of teeth and affect the development of the jaw and palate, leading to the need for orthodontic treatment. It's important for parents to address these habits early on and to seek advice from a paediatric dentist or orthodontist to prevent potential dental and orthodontic problems later on.

HOW CAN I TELL IF MY CHILD NEEDS ORTHODONTIC TREATMENT?

As a paediatric dentist, I often advise parents to look out for certain signs that their child may need orthodontic treatment. One such sign is if the child's smile appears very adult-like, with little spacing between the teeth. Ideally, children should have spacing between their teeth, unlike adults. Crowding, in the primary dentition, is a red flag. The reason why spacing is important is because the width of the permanent teeth that replace the primary teeth are larger. So an absence of spacing tends to result in crowding when the permanent teeth erupt.

Another indication that orthodontics may be needed is if there are discrepancies in the growth of the jaws, such as an underbite where the lower jaw is growing faster, or, if the upper arch is growing faster than the lower arch, resulting in a condition known as excessive overjet. These issues can be addressed with orthodontic intervention.

WHAT ARE THE BENEFITS OF DENTAL SEALANTS FOR CHILDREN?

Dental sealants are a type of polymer coating applied to the teeth to prevent bacteria and food debris from accumulating in the grooves. They create a barrier on the surface of the teeth, which reduces the risk of cavities. However, sealants can wear down over time and require periodic touch-ups, usually every three to six years.

2.2 - PREVENTION

by Dr. PAUL DOMINIQUE FROM USA

HOW CAN I PREPARE MY CHILD FOR THEIR FIRST DENTAL VISIT?

When parents ask me how to prepare their child for their first dental visit, I suggest that they start by discussing the upcoming visit with their child in a positive and reassuring manner. It's important to normalize the experience and let the child know that visiting the dentist is a regular part of maintaining good oral health. You can read children's books or watch videos that show children having positive dental experiences to help alleviate any fear or anxiety. It's also a good idea to schedule the appointment during a time when the child is well-rested and not hungry to minimize any potential discomfort or fussiness.

HOW CAN I HELP MY CHILD OVERCOME THEIR FEAR OF THE DENTIST?

One strategy to help children feel more comfortable during their first dental visit is to schedule a desensitizing appointment beforehand. This allows the child to become familiar with the dental office and the staff without undergoing any procedures. During this appointment, the child can observe and explore the environment in a non-threatening way. Not all paediatric dentists offer desensitizing appointments, so it's important to ask if this option is available. By normalizing the dental experience and making the child feel at ease, the first visit can set a positive tone for future dental appointments.

HOW CAN I PREPARE MY CHILD FOR A DENTAL PROCEDURE?

Preparing a child for a dental procedure can be a daunting task, but there are steps that can be taken to make the experience less stressful. It's important to communicate with your child in an age-appropriate manner about what to expect during the procedure. Avoid using scary or negative language that could increase their anxiety. Instead, focus on the positive aspects of maintaining healthy teeth and gums. One effective approach is to involve the dental professional in the preparation process. Ask the dentist or dental hygienist to explain the procedure to your child in a gentle and reassuring manner. They have the training and experience to answer questions and address any concerns your child may have.

Another helpful tip is to use play therapy or role-playing to familiarise your child with the procedure. This can help them understand what will happen during the visit and alleviate any fears they may have. Additionally, bringing a comfort item such as a stuffed animal or favourite toy can help your child feel more at ease during the appointment. In summary, preparing a child for a dental procedure requires a gentle and reassuring approach. Communication, involvement of the dental professional, and role-playing therapy can all be effective tools to reduce anxiety and create a positive experience for your child.

IS IT OKAY FOR CHILDREN TO CONSUME SUGARY FOODS AND DRINKS?

Consuming foods and drinks that are high in fermentable carbohydrates and sugars can increase the risk of developing dental caries. These include sugary snacks, candy, soda, and fruit juices. The bacteria in the mouth feed on these substances and produce acid, which can erode tooth enamel and lead to decay. It is important to limit the frequency of consuming these types of foods and drinks, and to practice good oral hygiene, such as brushing twice a day and flossing daily, to reduce the risk of developing dental caries.

CAN MY CHILD STILL ENJOY SWEET TREATS WHILE MAINTAINING GOOD ORAL HYGIENE?

When it comes to sugary drinks, it's important to be mindful of how they affect children's oral health. While it's okay for kids to have treats occasionally, parents should avoid putting sugary beverages in sippy cups that allow the child to constantly sip on them throughout the day. This prolonged exposure to sugar can give bacteria in the mouth the time they need to metabolize it into acid, which can lead to dental cavities. Instead, parents should give sugary drinks in small cups and encourage the child to finish it in one sitting. If possible, rinsing the mouth or brushing the teeth after consuming sugary drinks and snacks is also recommended to minimize the risk of tooth decay.

HOW CAN I ENSURE MY CHILD IS RECEIVING ADEQUATE NUTRITION FOR HEALTHY TEETH?

To ensure your child maintains good oral hygiene, it's important to focus on their diet. Encourage them to eat a diet high in fresh vegetables and fruits, and low in fermentable carbohydrates and processed foods. These foods can cause dental caries as they leave residue on the teeth that bacteria in the plaque metabolize into acid, which attacks the enamel. While it may be difficult to limit sweet treats, it's crucial to do so as much as possible. Along with a healthy diet, it's important to ensure your child is brushing and flossing adequately to remove plaque from their teeth. Mechanical debridement (removal with the bristles of a toothbrush) of the plaque is essential for good oral hygiene.

Regarding the myth about cheese and milk being good for teeth, it's important to note that once teeth are formed, they have already received the necessary amount of calcium. However, maintaining a diet high in calcium is crucial for overall health. Some parents are opting for a dairy-free diet for their children, and recent evidence suggests that alternative sources of calcium, such as green leafy vegetables and chia seeds, may be very effective.

HOW CAN I ENSURE MY CHILD IS GETTING ENOUGH FLUORIDE?
While most children today are getting an adequate amount of fluoride, there is a growing concern about overexposure leading to fluorosis, which can cause teeth to become brittle and prone to cavities. In cases where children are unable to spit out toothpaste, it is recommended to use a non-fluoridated option. It's worth noting that even if a community's water is not fluoridated, many popular beverages still contain fluoride. Overuse of fluoride, often prescribed by paediatricians, can lead to cosmetic issues such as hypomineralised areas on the teeth. These lesions can be susceptible to dental decay requiring filling or even stainless steel crowns.

HOW CAN I PREVENT ORTHODONTIC PROBLEMS IN MY CHILD?
Orthodontic issues in children involve several factors, including genetics, tooth eruption patterns, and oral habits. While genetics and tooth development are largely out of our control, we can reduce the risk of orthodontic problems by addressing harmful oral

habits. These habits include thumb-sucking, pacifier use, tongue-thrusting, and mouth-breathing. Parents should be aware of these habits and work with their children to eliminate them early on to avoid the need for extensive orthodontic treatment in the future. Regular dental check-ups can also help identify any issues early on and interceptive orthodontic therapy can be accomplished to mitigate the need for more extensive and expensive treatment later on.

2.3 - TIME

by Dr. PAUL DOMINIQUE FROM USA

WHAT IS THE BEST AGE FOR A CHILD TO START SEEING A DENTIST?

To ensure the best oral health for children, paediatric dentists recommend scheduling a dental visit as soon as the first teeth erupt into the mouth, which typically are the lower mandibular incisors. These teeth typically appear around six months of age. This early visit helps to establish a dental home for the child and allows them to become comfortable with the dental experience from a young age. During the first appointment, parents can receive guidance on how to properly care for their child's teeth and receive nutritional advice to support good oral health.

Although this is the typical recommendation, there are situations where children may need to see a dentist earlier. For example, some children are born with natal teeth which can pose a risk for aspiration and require prompt removal. In these cases, local anesthesia and specialized paediatric dental forceps are needed to safely remove the teeth. As a paediatric dentist, I recently saw a newborn, just two days after birth, to remove natal teeth, at the request of a neonatologist, due to the risks of aspiration and to ensure the mother can breastfeed comfortably.

HOW OFTEN SHOULD MY CHILD SEE A DENTIST?

To maintain good oral health, it's recommended to visit the dentist every six months, especially from around age three when the entire dentition has erupted. These regular visits help to identify any issues early on and allow for timely intervention and treatment. By staying on top of dental appointments, parents can help ensure their child's teeth and gums stay healthy and prevent potential complications in the future.

WHAT IS THE BEST AGE FOR A CHILD TO GET ORTHODONTIC TREATMENT?

To ensure optimal orthodontic treatment, it's important to start early as possible and not wait until all permanent teeth have erupted. Starting earlier allows for the orthodontist to work with growth and development and make actual orthopedic or skeletal changes that cannot be made later in adolescence. Typically, when a child has their four maxillary and four mandibular incisors and their permanent six-year molars, both maxillary and mandibular, it's a good time to start comprehensive orthodontic treatment with phase one. However, every child is different, and treatment may be required earlier or later than this timeframe, depending on their unique condition.

In some cases, parents may hear from certain orthodontists who don't like to work with children that it's better to wait until all permanent teeth have erupted before starting orthodontic treatment. However, in the experience of many dental professionals, starting earlier has many advantages. By changing the supporting bone structure that houses the teeth at an earlier age, there is less relapse and a more stable treatment outcome. While starting earlier may result in longer treatment time with both phase one and phase two, it's worth it in the long run to achieve the best results. Both paediatric dentists and orthodontists are qualified to perform early orthodontic treatment, and in some cases, a combination of both may be employed for the best results. The decision of who will perform the treatment will depend on the type of practice and the expertise of the dental professionals involved.

WHAT ARE THE SIGNS OF TEETH ERUPTION IN A CHILD?

When teeth are erupting, you may notice swelling in the alveolus, which is the bony ridge that supports the teeth. This swelling may appear blue or purple and is called an eruption hematoma. As the teeth migrate towards the epithelium (gum tissue), the epithelium may start to thin out and become translucent. You may even be able to see the imprints of the teeth during this process.

2.4 - MAINTENANCE

by Dr. PAUL DOMINIQUE FROM USA

WHAT IS THE RIGHT WAY TO CLEAN MY CHILD'S TEETH?

It is not enough to assume that children who regularly visit the dentist will not develop cavities. To prevent cavities, we need to monitor the children's oral hygiene practices. Our plan is to identify children in daycare centres who may be at risk for developing cavities by sampling their oral microbiota. We can then intervene early by providing aggressive preventive care, including frequent professional debridement. Unlike other medical conditions, dentistry has the unique advantage of being able to provide hands-on care by removing plaque directly from the patient's teeth.

HOW CAN I ENCOURAGE MY CHILD TO BRUSH THEIR TEETH REGULARLY?

To ensure good oral hygiene for children, it is recommended to clean their teeth from a young age. Lying them on a flat surface, with their mouth facing upwards, can be an effective method. Using a soft toothbrush with a small head, parents can adequately debride plaque off their child's teeth without the need for toothpaste. It is important to focus on all five surfaces of the teeth, including the chewing surface, the surface facing the lips/ cheeks, the surface facing the tongue, and the two surfaces in between. Parents should continue to clean their child's teeth until they have developed adequate hand-eye coordination, which typically occurs around nine years of age.

In terms of brushing time, the standard recommendation is two minutes in the morning and two minutes at night, totalling four minutes a day. However, the more important factor is to brush until all teeth have been adequately cleaned and debrided of any plaque, which may take longer than two minutes for some children. To encourage regular brushing, parents can make it a fun and interactive experience by using colourful toothbrushes and toothpaste with their child's favourite character. Additionally, parents can lead by example and brush their teeth with their children, making it a bonding experience. Rewards can also be given for consistent brushings, such as stickers or a special treat. It is important to make brushing a positive experience rather than a chore.

HOW CAN I PREVENT TOOTH DECAY IN MY CHILD'S BABY TEETH?

To promote good oral health for your child, it's important to focus on their diet and reduce their exposure to sugary beverages. A diet that is low in fermentable carbohydrates and unprocessed foods is ideal. Additionally, it's important to limit the amount of time your child spends with a bottle or sippy cup, especially at bedtime, as this can lead to nursing bottle caries. While milk is a good source of calcium, it also contains lactose, a naturally occurring sugar that can become cariogenic (cavity-causing) if there's prolonged exposure to the teeth' surfaces. So, while it's fine for your child to drink milk, it's important to limit their intake and make sure they don't drink it for extended periods of time. In other words, have them consume the milk in one sitting in a regular cup and not in a bottle or soppy cup which increases the time the milk makes contact with the teeth.

HOW CAN I PREVENT MY CHILD FROM DEVELOPING DENTAL ANXIETY?

When parents reference dentistry in casual conversation with children, it's important NOT to speak negatively about the experience or share scary stories. Instead, normalize it as a regular part of life and emphasize that the dentist is there to help them. It's important to avoid making a big deal out of dental appointments and not to create unnecessary fear or anxiety in the child. By presenting dentistry in a positive light and highlighting the benefits of good oral health, children are more likely to view dental visits as a routine part of their healthcare.

HOW CAN I HELP MY CHILD AVOID DENTAL INJURIES?

To prevent dental injuries for children who are active in sports, it is recommended to see a dentist or orthodontist to have a sports guard made. It is especially important for children with a discrepancy in their teeth, such as an overjet or "buck teeth," to consult with an orthodontist. Research has shown that children with a more severe overjet are more likely to have injuries to their incisors. In addition to a sports guard, it is important to counsel children on safety measures and remind them that what is safe for the rest of the body is also safe for their teeth.

HOW CAN I HELP MY CHILD AVOID GUM DISEASE?

Fortunately, advanced gum disease is not very common in children, but plaque-associated gingivitis can frequently occur. Adequate brushing is the best way to prevent gingivitis, ensuring that the child is using the proper technique to remove plaque from the teeth and under the gum line. Flossing is also beneficial and should be introduced as soon as there are tight contacts between the teeth, usually when the child is older and has less spacing between their teeth. It's important to show the child how to properly floss and to make it a regular part of their oral hygiene routine.

HOW CAN I HELP MY CHILD MAINTAIN GOOD ORAL HYGIENE WHILE WEARING BRACES?
To maintain good oral health, it is important to prioritize adequate brushing, a healthy diet, and warm salt water rinses. However, when a child has braces, it can be challenging to properly clean around the brackets, and parental supervision is necessary to ensure proper brushing techniques and the use of adjuncts such as floss threaders or super floss. Additionally, an electric toothbrush can be helpful, but it ultimately depends on how well it is used.

HOW CAN I HELP MY CHILD AVOID TOOTH SENSITIVITY?
Tooth sensitivity is a common problem among teenagers, and it's caused by porous enamel and odontoblastic processes that make teeth more sensitive to hot and cold sensations. One way to help children avoid sensitivity is to use toothpaste specifically designed for sensitive teeth, which contains potassium nitrate. This ingredient stabilizes the odontoblastic processes and reduces their sensitivity to temperature changes.

However, it's important to ensure that children do not swallow toothpaste, especially medicated ones like those for sensitive teeth, as they contain ingredients like sodium fluoride and potassium nitrate that can be harmful if ingested over time. Additionally, when children have braces, parents should supervise their brushing to ensure that all the brackets are adequately cleaned, and they may need to use adjuncts like floss threaders or super floss to clean between wires and brackets. Overall, a combination of adequate brushing, nutritional excellence, and warm salt water rinses can help prevent tooth sensitivity and other dental issues in children.

2.5 - DENTAL WORK

by Dr. PAUL DOMINIQUE FROM USA 🇺🇸

WHAT ARE THE MOST COMMON DENTAL PROBLEMS IN CHILDREN?

One of the most prevalent issues I come across in children is dental caries or cavities. Surprisingly, it's seven times more common than asthma.

WHAT CAN I DO IF MY CHILD HAS A DENTAL EMERGENCY?

It's important to note that hospitals typically do not have dental personnel available around the clock, and therefore may not be equipped to handle urgent dental issues. It's always best to try to schedule an appointment with a paediatric dentist or general dentist during regular business hours, and if the emergency happens after hours, then going to the emergency room may be necessary, but keep in mind that dental care may not be readily available.

IS IT NECESSARY FOR MY CHILD TO HAVE DENTAL X-RAYS TAKEN?

The American Dental Association recommends that a child's first dental visit should occur within six months of the first tooth erupting, but routine dental X-rays are not usually taken until the child is at least 2-3 years old. X-rays are usually taken to look for dental cavities between the teeth, as it's not possible for the dentist to identify cavities between the teeth by visual inspection. It's important to note that today's modern dental X-rays are not a significant source of radiation exposure, and are safe.

WHAT IS THE BEST WAY TO TREAT A CHILD'S CAVITIES?

When it comes to treating dental cavities in children, there is no one-size-fits-all solution. The approach depends on various factors, such as the severity of the cavity and the type of tooth affected. For small lesions in a single tooth, a treatment called silver diamine fluoride (SDF) can arrest the cavity's progression. However, SDF does not reverse the damage or restore the tooth's structure. For very small cavities on anterior teeth, tooth-coloured fillings could be used to restore these teeth after the cavity is removed.

With extensive cavities, on anterior teeth, traditional fillings may not be the best option due to the inherent limitations of the tooth-coloured filling material. Instead, dentists may use aesthetic caps or crowns to restore the tooth's appearance and function. For posterior teeth with conservative cavities, tooth-coloured restorations or amalgam fillings may suffice. However, if the cavity is too large, a stainless steel crown or aesthetic crown may be necessary.

In some cases, general anesthesia or IV sedation may be required to treat multiple cavities or if the child is uncooperative. These procedures usually take place in a hospital but can be in office in conjunction with a medical anesthesiologist. It's worth noting that prevention is always better than cure. Encouraging good oral hygiene habits, such as brushing and flossing, and limiting sugary foods and drinks can reduce the risk of dental cavities in children.

WHAT IS DENTAL SEALANT, AND IS IT NECESSARY FOR MY CHILD?

It's important to note that dental sealants are not a one-size-fits-all solution. Research shows that they have a good track record only on certain teeth, specifically the six-year and twelve-year molars. On premolars and primary teeth, they do not hold up as well. Therefore, it's important to consult with your child's dentist to determine if dental sealants are appropriate for their specific teeth. While they are not necessary, they can be beneficial in maintaining good oral health when used on the appropriate teeth.

WHAT ARE THE BENEFITS OF ORTHODONTIC TREATMENT FOR CHILDREN?

There are a variety of benefits to orthodontic treatment, ranging from cosmetic to functional. On the cosmetic side, having straight teeth can improve a child's self-esteem and confidence. On the functional side, orthodontic treatment can address jaw growth discrepancies and prevent future jaw joint issues. Early intervention can modify growth and prevent more severe issues down the line. Overall, orthodontic treatment can have both immediate and long-term benefits for a child's oral health and overall well-being.

IS IT OKAY FOR MY CHILD TO PLAY SPORTS WITH BRACES?

It is possible for children to engage in sports activities even with braces, but it's important to keep in mind that braces may increase the risk of soft tissue injuries, particularly to the lips. However, braces can also be advantageous in certain cases of dental injuries, like when a child experiences significant trauma to the teeth. Braces can provide stability to the affected teeth and act as a splint, much like how a helmet safeguards the head. When it comes to sports and braces, every situation is unique. Therefore, it's crucial for parents to consult with their dentist to determine the best course of action. By doing so, they can ensure that their child can enjoy playing sports while minimizing the risk of dental injuries.

WHAT ARE THE RISKS OF NOT TREATING MY CHILD'S CAVITIES?

When a child's cavities are not treated, the tooth's demineralization process can continue, potentially causing the cavity to become deeper and reach the nerve of the tooth, which may result in pain, infection, and even death in very rare instances. Furthermore, untreated cavities may require extraction, leading to difficulties with eating and speaking. Children may experience pain, discomfort, and sensitivity from cavities, which can impact their daily lives. Cavities can also cause damage and decay to surrounding teeth and lead to tooth loss, resulting in long-term consequences for their oral health, speech, and self-esteem.

Delaying treatment for cavities can result in costly dental treatments, such as root canals, crowns, and extractions, which can be more extensive and expensive in the future. Seeking treatment for your child's cavities is crucial to prevent further damage and potential complications.

HOW CAN I PREVENT BABY BOTTLE TOOTH DECAY IN MY CHILD?

Baby bottle tooth decay is a common condition that occurs when the teeth of young children are frequently exposed to sugary liquids, such as milk, juice, or formula, for extended periods. This exposure can lead to the demineralization of the teeth, causing decay, pain, and potential infection. To prevent baby bottle tooth decay, it is essential to limit the consumption of sugary liquids and adopt good oral hygiene practices early on. Avoid putting your child to bed with a bottle or letting them walk around with a bottle or sip cup, as this can prolong the exposure to sugary liquids and increase the risk of decay. Instead, offer the bottle during meal times only and encourage the child to drink from a cup as soon as they are able to do so

In addition, it is crucial to clean your child's teeth and gums regularly, starting from the time their first tooth appears. Use a soft-bristled brush and water or a non-fluoridated toothpaste, depending on the child's age and dental needs. Regular dental check-ups and cleanings can also help detect and prevent decay before it becomes severe. By following these simple but effective preventive measures, parents can help protect their child's teeth and ensure optimal oral health in the long run.

HOW CAN I FIND A PAEDIATRIC DENTIST FOR MY CHILD?

To find a good paediatric dentist, start by checking the American Academy of Paediatric Dentists website or the Canadian Academy of Paediatric Dentistry. They have resources to help you locate a dentist in your area. Once you have a list of potential dentists, you can read online reviews, but keep in mind that some reviews may be biased or unhelpful. To assess reviews effectively, look for patterns in the feedback and pay attention to comments about the dentist's communication style and chair-side manner. You can also ask friends or family members for recommendations. All qualified paediatric dentists have completed an accredited residency program and are qualified to provide dental care to children. When you find a good dentist, stick with them to ensure your child receives consistent and high-quality care.

HOW CAN I HELP MY CHILD MAINTAIN GOOD ORAL HYGIENE WHILE WEARING APPLIANCES?

It's important to supervise your child's oral hygiene routine. One helpful tool is disclosing tablets, which can be purchased online and stain the plaque on teeth to make it visible for easy monitoring. Simply remove the colourized plaque until the tooth is visible again. This method can be used with appliances as well.

2.6 - FEAR/PAIN
by Dr. PAUL DOMINIQUE FROM USA

IS SEDATION DENTISTRY NECESSARY FOR CHILDREN?

When it comes to sedation during dental procedures, it's important to prioritize your child's safety. Dental instruments can be dangerous, so sedation may be necessary if your child has severe dental disease or a condition that could worsen and cause pain or infection. Sedation comes in three forms: oral sedation, intravenous (IV) sedation, and general anesthesia at a hospital. Oral sedation involves the dentist giving your child a mild sedative agent or cocktail of agents to reduce anxiety, often combined with nitrous oxide. However, this method is the least beneficial and least predictable due to the unpredictability of drug absorption. Many paediatric dentists are moving away from offering oral sedation.

IV sedation, on the other hand, is very effective and safe when administered by a medical anesthesiologist who specializes in paediatric anesthesia. The anesthesiologist provides a short-acting anesthetic agent that can be titrated to achieve the desired effect. However, not every child is a candidate for IV sedation, especially if they have a complex medical condition. The safest method of sedation is general anesthesia in a hospital setting, especially for children with complex medical issues or those who are very young and cannot be safely sedated in the office. This method involves the use of an inhaled gas to induce anesthesia, followed by IV administration. The advantage of this method is that the airway is managed through the insertion of a breathing tube, ensuring optimal safety for your child.

In summary, sedation should only be used when necessary, and the best method of sedation depends on your child's individual situation. It's important to discuss these options with your child's primary healthcare provider and paediatric dentist to determine the best course of action for your child.

HOW CAN I HELP MY CHILD COPE WITH TOOTH LOSS?

Tooth loss can be an emotional experience for children, especially if it's their first time. One thing you can do to help them cope is to acknowledge their feelings and reassure them that it's normal to feel a bit scared or unsure. You can also explain the tooth loss process to them and how it's a sign that they're growing up. To make it fun, consider creating a tooth fairy tradition where they can leave their lost tooth under their pillow for a special treat or reward. Finally, it's important to encourage good dental hygiene habits and explain how taking care of their teeth can help prevent future tooth loss.

HOW CAN I RELIEVE MY CHILD'S TOOTH ERUPTION PAIN?

In terms of tooth eruption pain, I would suggest using children's Tylenol as it is a safe and effective pain reliever. While some parents may be tempted to use over-the-counter remedies with topical aesthetics, these can actually burn the gingiva and cause irritation once the anesthetic wears off. Another option that some parents find helpful is using chewable devices that can be frozen and then chewed on for the cold sensation, which can also provide some relief.

WHAT ARE THE RISKS OF USING TEETHING GELS AND CREAMS?

While it is true that teething gels and creams can cause gingival irritation, there are other potential risks as well. Overdosing or poisoning is possible if the product is used excessively or if it contains ingredients that are harmful in large amounts, such as benzocaine. It is important to follow the instructions on the packaging carefully and to consult with a healthcare provider if there are any concerns.

HOW CAN I HELP MY CHILD RECOVER AFTER A DENTAL PROCEDURE?

There are a few issues that children may experience immediately after a dental procedure, particularly related to local anesthesia. When the procedure is done, the child's lips may feel numb, which can be an unpleasant experience for them. Parents should reassure their child that this is temporary and that the sensation will come back soon. It's also important to be vigilant, as the child may accidentally bite their lip or tongue due to the lack of feeling. Typically, the local anesthetic lasts for a few hours, and parents can tell their child that it will wear off after the length of two Disney movies or by the time the second movie is done. While there are agents available to reverse the effect of local anesthesia and bring back feeling quicker, they are not currently approved for use in children.

2.7 - MONEY

by Dr. PAUL DOMINIQUE FROM USA

WHAT IS THE COST OF PAEDIATRIC DENTAL CARE?

While it's true that children's dental procedures tend to be less complex than adult procedures, it's important to note that there are still differences in the cost of treatment between children and adults. Children's dentistry may be less expensive than adult dentistry due to the nature of the procedures, but it's not necessarily true that there is no significant difference between the cost of filling an adult tooth versus a child's tooth. It's also important to keep in mind that the cost of dental treatment can vary greatly depending on factors such as location, type of procedure, and individual dental practice pricing.

ARE THOSE COVERED BY THE GOVERNMENT?

In the USA, the administration of Medicaid varies by state in the United States, with federal funds being allocated to each state for the program. However, how the funds are spent is at the discretion of the states, and some states allocate more funding toward children's dentistry than others. In Georgia, for example, Medicaid coverage for children is good, but in states like Florida, coverage is poor, resulting in a shortage of dentists who accept Medicaid insurance for children.

ARE INSURANCE COVERING CHILD DENTAL CARE?

Some private insurance plans in the USA may cover children's dental services, but the extent of coverage and requirements for accessing care may vary depending on the insurance provider and state of residence. It is important to check with your insurance provider to understand what services are covered and any associated costs or limitations.

2.8 - HABITS

by Dr. PAUL DOMINIQUE FROM USA

IS THUMB-SUCKING HARMFUL TO MY CHILD'S TEETH?

Thumb sucking can be harmful to a child's dental health. The pressure created by the sucking action, combined with the thumb being in the mouth, can affect the bony supporting structure or alveolus in the mouth. If thumb sucking is allowed to continue, it can result in permanent changes to the dental arch. In some cases, braces may be necessary to restore the normal architecture of the dental arch. Therefore, it's important to discourage thumb-sucking in children to prevent potential dental problems later on.

HOW CAN I ENCOURAGE MY CHILD TO STOP THUMB-SUCKING?

There are several ways to help children stop thumb-sucking. For younger children, one effective method is to use a solution that can be painted on the digit they are sucking on, making it taste sour and unappealing. Devices can also be used to discourage the habit, such as rubbing the digit or being firm when the child is caught sucking their thumb. If the habit persists into older ages, customized dental appliances can be made to prevent thumb-sucking or tongue-thrusting. These can include shields that prevent the digit m from entering the mouth or stopping the tongue from being thrust forward. The Bluegrass Appliance, which uses a suspended bead to encourage the patient's tongue to play with the bead instead of thumb sucking or tongue thrusting.

HOW CAN I PREVENT MY CHILD FROM GRINDING THEIR TEETH AT NIGHT?

There are currently no proven methods to stop nocturnal grinding during nighttime as it is a subconscious behavioural habit. Although parents may hear the grinding from adjacent rooms, it is difficult to treat, as it is outside of the child's conscious awareness. However, some psychologists can provide exercises, done during the day. to reduce grinding at night, such as blowing air between the teeth. It is believed that stress can cause grinding, and studies have shown that children who experience stressful situations, such as the parents getting divorced, changing schools etc; grind their teeth more frequently than children who do not experience these stressors.

WHAT ARE THE DANGERS OF SHARING UTENSILS AND DRINKS WITH MY CHILD?
Sharing utensils and drinks with a child can transmit harmful bacteria and viruses, including those that cause dental caries. While it's true that children can acquire their mother's oral microbiome early on in life, it's still important to be cautious with other caregivers or individuals with dental disease. HSV-1 or herpes simplex-1 while it's a common infection, that affects 90% of the population in the US and globally. HSV-1 can be spread through close contact with infected individuals, there is evidence to suggest that grandmothers are the primary source of transmission. It's important to practice good hygiene and avoid sharing utensils or engaging in close contact with individuals who have active HSV-1 lesions or fever blisters.

HOW CAN I HELP MY CHILD AVOID JAW PROBLEMS?
When you refer to jaw problems, I assume this refers to issues relating to jaw growth differential, resulting in skeletal class III or class II occlusion. It's important to understand that some jaw problems can be congenital and genetically programmed. While there may not be a lot you can do to prevent your child from having jaw problems, there are certain parafunctional habits that can exacerbate them. For example, lower jaw thrusting can encourage growth in the lower jaw and create a discrepancy in growth between the upper and lower

jaw. Therefore, it's important to encourage your child not to engage in any parafunctional habits to avoid worsening of jaw issues.

HOW CAN I PREVENT DENTAL PROBLEMS IN MY CHILD WHILE THEY ARE SLEEPING?

Preventing dental problems in children requires being mindful of their habits, particularly when it comes to sleeping habits. One simple step parents can take is to avoid giving their children sugary beverages in a bottle while they sleep. Additionally, parents should ensure that their child is breathing properly through their nostrils, as mouth breathing can cause jaw issues and a constricted palate. A paediatrician or ENT doctor can provide guidance on this matter. Mouth breathing can also lead to dry mouth and an increased risk of dental caries, so proper breathing is essential for oral health. By being proactive in these ways, parents can help reduce the risk of dental problems in their children.

This is **ALPHA DENTISTRY vol. 3, PAEDIATRIC DENTISTRY FAQ**. Welcome to the Alphas.

Dr. BAK NGUYEN

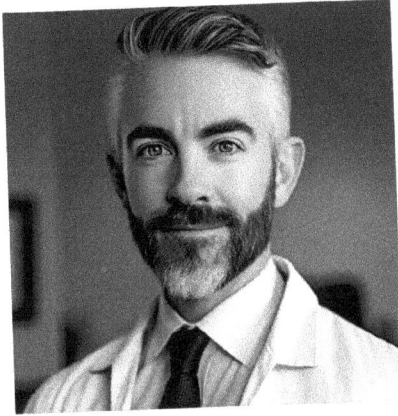

Dr. RICHARD SIMPSON,
DMD

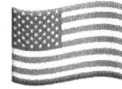

From the USA, **Dr. RICHARD SIMPSON**, DMD, is a board-certified paediatric dentist in private practice and a veteran with 15 years of military service. Dr. Simpson is a Diplomate in the American Board of Paediatric Dentistry, and a Fellow in The American College of Dentists, the International College of Dentists, and the American Academy of Pediatric Dentistry. He has held numerous health professional leadership positions and has experience in state and national cross-sector networking, telehealth/teledentistry, child advocacy, health disparities, policy, and advancing improved medical-dental integration and access to care. He is skilled in leadership, project design and implementation, advocacy, and inter-professional and public-private collaboration. He believes that telehealth is the integral to the future of dentistry and the oral health-overall healthcare paradigm. Dr Simpson is the Immediate Past-Chair of the Oral Health Coalition of Alabama, He serves as and has recently completed his tenure as the Chief Clinical Officer for Holland Healthcare, an international telehealth oral imaging innovator. Dr. Simpson is a member of the Advisory Boards of The TeleDentists and Soluria He and he serves as a Thought Leader and collaborator with TeethCloud, a global oral health initiative dedicated to reducing oral health inequities through technology and DI. Dr. Simpson was recently selected to the 2023 Class of the World's Top 100 Doctors by members of the Global Summits Institute.

Richard and I met in the field, in the midst of the action, in the COVID pandemic. Both of us were looking for a solution and we met as tele-dentistry was a proposed solution to resume our function, back in the Spring of 2020.

Through online interactions, we spotted one another. It is funny how it is often the same people you meet as you are actively involved. This is how we gained each other respect and started a friendship.

When I invited Dr. Simpson to join the Alphas as a co-author. That was a year prior to the beginning of the book. Very quickly, he started recruiting paediatric dentists to join the team. We've become great friends since, even if I keep calling him sir (lol)!

Dr. Simpson is much more than a dentist. He is a gentleman, a true friend, and the kind of partner to have as you are trying to change the world for the better. Citizen of the Year, Top100 Doc are a few of Dr. Simpson's awards and titles. Well, to me, he is a great friend, a respected doctor, and an Alpha.

Without further ado, please join me to welcome Dr. Richard Simpson.

This is **ALPHA DENTISTRY vol. 3, PAEDIATRIC DENTISTRY FAQ**.
Welcome to the Alphas.

Dr. BAK NGUYEN

CHAPTER 3

"PAEDIATRIC DENTISTRY"

by Dr. RICHARD SIMPSON

FROM USA 🇺🇸

3.1 - DEFINITIONS

by Dr. RICHARD SIMPSON FROM USA

WHAT IS THE BEST TYPE OF TOOTHBRUSH FOR MY CHILD?

When choosing a toothbrush for a child, it's best to go with a soft or medium bristle brush that's appropriate for their age. Different sizes are available, ranging from infant to adult, so make sure to select one that's small enough to fit comfortably in the child's mouth and allow for proper brushing technique. The ADA Seal of Approval is a good indication of quality, as it signifies that the brush has been tested and shown to be effective.

As for electric toothbrushes, they can be a useful tool for some children, especially those who struggle with manual brushing due to coordination issues or special needs. Electric brushes take the action out of the wrist and put it in the head, making it easier to reach all areas of the mouth. Some models even come with features that make brushing more fun for children, such as lights or music.

That being said, both manual and electric toothbrushes can be efficient when used properly. The choice ultimately depends on the child's needs and preferences. If a child consistently shows poor hygiene despite manual brushing, an electric brush may be worth trying as a motivational or efficiency-enhancing tool.

WHAT IS THE ROLE OF FLUORIDE IN PREVENTING CAVITIES?

Fluoride is an important mineral that helps strengthen the enamel of our teeth. Throughout the day, our mouths experience a decrease in pH and an increase in acid every time we eat or drink. As a result, minerals are released from the enamel on a microscopic level and then reabsorbed as the pH returns to neutral. It is important that this "demineralization" and "remineralization" remains in balance. If there are frequent or prolonged periods of low pH or high acidity, we lose more minerals than we can replace, which can lead to tooth decay. By incorporating fluoride into the enamel, it can help provide additional resistance against mineral loss, along with other minerals such as calcium and phosphates.

WHAT IS THE DIFFERENCE BETWEEN A PAEDIATRIC DENTIST AND A GENERAL DENTIST?

A paediatric dentist is a dental specialist who provides dental care to infants, children, adolescents, and individuals with special needs. Unlike a general dentist who may provide care to patients of all ages, a paediatric dentist has completed additional training, typically two to three years, in the specialty of paediatric dentistry. This specialized training allows them to provide age-appropriate care, manage behaviour, and address the unique dental needs of children, including those with medical or developmental conditions. Paediatric dentists are also trained to provide dental care in hospital settings and work with other healthcare professionals to provide comprehensive care. In addition to being dental specialists, paediatric dentists are also considered primary care providers, similar to paediatricians, as they are often the first line of defense in maintaining a child's oral health and wellness.

WHAT ARE THE MOST COMMON ORTHODONTIC PROBLEMS IN CHILDREN?

The biggest concern we hear from parents is often the lack of space for teeth to come in properly aligned, but there are various types of orthodontic problems that can be addressed at different stages of development. Orthodontic issues can be broadly divided into skeletal/facial problems related to the jaws and arch form, and dental problems related to tooth size, position, and angulation. Crowding is one of the most common issues we deal with, but we also focus on addressing orthodontic problems related to the relationship between the jaws, teeth, and face.

As paediatric dentists, we specialize in growth and development and monitor a child's development from infancy through adolescence. We are trained to intervene at certain stages, such as providing guidance for tooth eruption or addressing functional bite discrepancies like crossbites. Some paediatric dentists, like myself, have extensive additional orthodontic training and provide full-scope orthodontic care, while others work closely with orthodontists or refer all treatment needs to them. The American Orthodontic Association recommends an evaluation by age 7-8. As paediatric dentists, we consistently monitor a child's growth and development, enabling us to work closely with our orthodontist colleagues in determining when it's the best time to consider limited or comprehensive orthodontic treatment based on our level of expertise and practice preference.

HOW CAN I TELL IF MY CHILD NEEDS ORTHODONTIC TREATMENT?

It's important for parents to be aware of their child's oral health, but it's also important to recognize that there are many aspects of dental needs that may not be immediately visible to them. While parents may be able to notice issues like crowding or misaligned teeth, there are other problems that may require the expertise of a paediatric dentist or general dentist with experience in growth and development. As dental professionals, it's our role to inform parents of all aspects of their child's oral health and provide guidance on appropriate intervention, monitoring, and timing. This may include anticipating issues like crowding or impacted teeth and taking action to prevent more serious problems from developing in the future. By working closely with parents and patients, we can ensure that all aspects of their oral health are addressed and that we are providing the best possible care.

WHAT ARE THE BENEFITS OF DENTAL SEALANTS FOR CHILDREN?

Well, dental sealants are an important tool in preventing tooth decay, especially on the chewing surfaces of the back teeth which have grooves and pits that are difficult to clean. These areas can easily harbour bacteria and cause cavities, even with good hygiene and diet. Sealants are a protective coating that is applied to the teeth to seal these grooves and pits, preventing bacteria from settling in and blocking bacteria from food sources in the oral environment, thereby reducing the risk of cavities. However, not all children may require sealants.

Paediatric dentists typically conduct a risk assessment to determine a child's risk of decay based on factors such as their past history of decay, diet, hygiene practices, family history, and fluoride exposure. If a child is at a low risk of decay or has open and accessible fissures, then sealants may not be necessary. However, for children at moderate or high risk of decay or with well-defined grooves that are difficult to clean, sealants can be highly beneficial. Regular monitoring of the teeth can help identify any changes or areas that may require sealants in the future. Overall, sealants are an important preventive strategy for permanent molars, but their use should be assessed on a case-by-case basis.

3.2 - PREVENTION

by Dr. RICHARD SIMPSON FROM USA 🇺🇸

HOW CAN I PREPARE MY CHILD FOR THEIR FIRST DENTAL VISIT?

Firstly, it is important to note that the recommended age for a child's first dental visit is by age 1, according to major medical and dental organizations. For infants and toddlers, the visit is mainly an opportunity for the dentist to discuss any concerns, perform an oral health risk assessment, provide anticipatory guidance and preventive education to parents or caregivers, and administer fluoride varnish when indicated. Cleanings are not generally indicated at this age, and there is no expectation of cooperative behaviour for one or two-year-olds for these oral health well child visits.

For older children, around three to four years old, parents can take steps to prepare them for their dental visit. However, it is crucial to avoid passing on any anxious feelings or fears about the dentist to the child. Instead, parents should approach the visit with positivity and reassure the child that the dentist is someone who cares about their oral health and wants to help them achieve a beautiful, healthy smile. Parents can even get inexpensive mirrors to practice looking at and counting the teeth with their child. As the child grows older, parents can discuss the visit with them and encourage them to ask questions during the appointment.

HOW CAN I HELP MY CHILD OVERCOME THEIR FEAR OF THE DENTIST?

Well, the primary reason for dental anxiety in children can vary depending on their experiences and age. If they have not been to a dentist before, it's often fear of the unknown, fear of strangers, or fear based on what they have heard from others. However, if they have had a bad experience elsewhere, it can be a challenge to regain their confidence and reduce their fears. In such cases, it's essential to find out what their concerns are and reassure them that they are seeing someone who specializes in treating children. It's also important to work together as a team, involving the parents and dentist, to address the child's anxiety and build their confidence. As a paediatric dentist with almost thirty years of experience, I've learned that gaining a child's trust and building a rapport is the most significant factor in reducing anxiety, and the greatest challenge we face if the child has had a previous difficult experience elsewhere. However, with a positive approach and reassurance, we can help alleviate their fears and make their dental experience a positive one.

IS IT OKAY FOR CHILDREN TO CONSUME SUGARY FOODS AND DRINKS?

First, it's important to note that tooth decay, or 'bad teeth' as you sometimes hear, are not inherited, except in rare genetic disorders. It's caused by germs that use sugars and release acid, which then attacks the teeth. As a paediatric dentist, I always discuss with parents the importance of sugar intake and its effect on tooth decay. Frequent and prolonged exposure to sugars is a key factor in the development of cavities. While it's difficult to completely eliminate sugar from a child's diet, we should try to limit the frequency and duration of exposure. Sugary drinks and juices are a major culprit, especially when consumed between meals or at night, and sticky or sour substances can be particularly harmful to teeth. I try to offer alternatives such as sugarless gum or plain chocolate, which has been shown to dissolve quickly in the mouth and has some beneficial effects in reducing the damaging effects of the bacteria responsible for causing decay.

HOW CAN I ENSURE MY CHILD IS GETTING ENOUGH FLUORIDE?

Fluoride is naturally present in some foods grown in the ground, as well as naturally occurring in some water sources depending on where you live, but the most effective source of fluoride in preventing decay is through fluoridation of public water systems. This public health measure has been shown to reduce decay by up to 50% and is very cost-effective. Using fluoride toothpaste in combination with drinking fluoridated water provides adequate fluoride for many people who are otherwise at low risk for developing tooth decay. However, children who are at moderate or high risk of decay, due to factors such as poor dietary and hygiene practices, genetic defects, or a family history of decay, may require more frequent and targeted fluoride applications. Professional fluoride varnishes have been proven effective in reducing decay and remineralizing teeth, but their frequency of application should be determined based on the child's individual decay risk. Therefore, it is important to work with a paediatric dentist to identify the child's fluoride sources and decay risk and to determine the appropriate frequency of fluoride applications.

CAN MY CHILD STILL ENJOY SWEET TREATS WHILE MAINTAINING GOOD ORAL HYGIENE?

I think it's important to note that while maintaining good oral hygiene can certainly reduce the risk of tooth decay, it's not the only factor at play. Another critical factor is one's diet and sugar intake. Even with good oral hygiene practices, frequent consumption of sugary foods and drinks can still increase the risk of tooth decay. These two factors, hygiene and diet, are both important in determining an individual's risk for decay, but they are separate and distinct factors. It's essential to address both in order to maintain optimal oral health.

HOW CAN I PREVENT ORTHODONTIC PROBLEMS IN MY CHILD?

When it comes to preventing orthodontic problems in children, there are certain factors that cannot be prevented or controlled such as inherited facial growth patterns, jaw size, and tooth size. However, there are some things that parents can do at home to reduce the risk of orthodontic problems. For example, extended use of pacifiers can cause temporary effects on the front teeth, but if the habit is stopped before the second molars come in, the likelihood of having a crossbite can be reduced. Similarly, digit habits such as thumb or finger sucking can lead to orthodontic problems if they persist into permanent teeth, so it's important to work with a paediatric dentist to address these habits.

Good oral health is also important in preventing orthodontic problems, as tooth extractions or large cavities can cause crowding and impactions which can lead to more extensive orthodontic problems down the road. Early intervention, such as selective extractions or early correction of problems such as posterior or anterior crossbites with functional shifts can redirect permanent teeth and reduce the chance for impactions or reduce the extent of orthodontic problems. Overall, while not all orthodontic problems can be prevented, certain habits and early interventions can reduce the risk of problems developing or reduce the extent of treatment needed.

HOW CAN I PREPARE MY CHILD FOR A DENTAL PROCEDURE?

Preparing your child for a dental procedure can be a daunting task, but it's important to make sure they feel comfortable and prepared. First, it's important to choose a pediatric dentist who specializes in treating children and is skilled in communicating with them at their level. Next, although well-intentioned, sometimes too much explanation at home actually raises the level of concerns and anxiousness experienced by the child. Treatment procedures and approaches to child management for dental care have very positively evolved over the years, and parental experiences as a child are likely very different than the current care modalities.

Deferring the majority of explanation responsibilities to the experienced dental team is often the best approach, while demonstrating to your child your comfort and confidence in the dentist and his or her "helpers". We make sure to explain to your child what to expect during the procedure using age-appropriate language and avoiding scary or intimidating words. In advance, you can even ask the dentist for a simple explanation of what will happen so you can share it with your child before they return for the procedure. Additionally, encourage your child to ask questions and express any concerns they may have. Finally, bring comfort items such as a favourite stuffed animal or blanket to the appointment to help your child feel more at ease.

HOW CAN I ENSURE MY CHILD IS RECEIVING ADEQUATE NUTRITION FOR HEALTHY TEETH?
For a child's dental health, it's best to avoid introducing sugary substances at an early age to prevent developing a preference for sweets over healthier foods. Fruits are good for children, but fruit juices should be consumed in moderation. Children should be provided with a well balanced diet with adequate and varied protein sources, whole grains, fruits and vegetables, and healthy fats. Growing children need calcium and vitamin D for bone growth and density as well as proper development of permanent teeth that begin forming as early as age one. Parents should inform their pediatric dentist about any dietary restrictions, sensitivities, or allergies their child has so the dentist can recommend better ways to get necessary nutrients such as calcium and to reduce the number and duration of exposures to sweet substances. It's also important to establish good nutrition habits early and work with the pediatric dentist to promote good oral hygiene practices at home.

by Dr. RICHARD SIMPSON FROM USA 🇺🇸

WHAT IS THE BEST AGE FOR A CHILD TO START SEEING A DENTIST?

The American Academy of Pediatrics, American Academy of Pediatric Dentistry and the American Dental Association recommend that a child should have their first dental visit within six months of the eruption of the first tooth, or by the age of 12 months. This visit is treated as a well-child check for oral health. The majority of the visit is spent obtaining medical and dental history, assessing risk, discussing prevention and guidance, and examining the child. Applying fluoride varnish is a small part of the visit. The focus is on risk assessment and reducing risks through daily practices. Therefore, the age of one is the recommended time for a child's first dental visit.

HOW OFTEN SHOULD MY CHILD SEE A DENTIST?

There are different recommendations for dental check-ups depending on the child's age and risk level for dental issues. The traditional recommendation is to visit the dentist every six months, which can be useful for catching problems early and reinforcing positive experiences. However, for older children with low risk of decay and no history of problems, this frequency may not be necessary. On the other hand, high-risk children or those with early problems may need to be seen more often, sometimes as often as every three months, until the situation improves. Ultimately, the frequency of dental check-ups should be based on a risk assessment tailored to the child's specific needs.

WHAT IS THE BEST AGE FOR A CHILD TO GET ORTHODONTIC TREATMENT?

The symptoms and experiences associated with teething and tooth eruption can vary widely among children. Some may not exhibit any noticeable discomfort, while others may experience fussiness, agitation, increased salivation, and reduced hunger for a few days. It's important to note that teething does not follow a steady growth pattern and can occur in spurts. As for permanent molars, some children may complain of pain or discomfort when a new tooth is emerging, usually in the evenings or at night when growth hormone is increasing. It's also possible to see swelling or discolouration over a tooth before it emerges, which is typically nothing to worry about and resolves on its own.

When it comes to permanent teeth replacing baby teeth, discomfort and mobility are common. Sometimes children may experience pain when biting down due to the lessened structure of the baby tooth as the permanent tooth moves in. It's also possible to visually see changes in the tooth during this process such as when a baby tooth turns pinkish in color as it becomes thinner from resorption before it is lost.

WHAT ARE THE SIGNS OF TEETH ERUPTION IN A CHILD?

The symptoms and experiences associated with teething and tooth eruption can vary widely among children. Some may not exhibit any noticeable discomfort, while others may experience fussiness, agitation, increased salivation, and reduced hunger for a few days. It's important to note that teething does not follow a steady growth pattern and can occur in spurts. As for permanent molars, some children may complain of pain or discomfort when a new tooth is emerging, usually in the evenings or at night when growth hormone is increasing. It's also possible to see swelling or discolouration over a tooth before it emerges, which is typically nothing to worry about and resolves on its own.

When it comes to permanent teeth replacing baby teeth, discomfort and mobility are common. Sometimes children may experience pain when biting down due to the lessened structure of the baby tooth as the permanent tooth moves in. It's also possible to visually see changes in the tooth during this process such as when a baby tooth turns pinkish in colour as it becomes thinner from resorption before it is lost.

3.4 - MAINTENANCE

by Dr. RICHARD SIMPSON FROM USA

WHAT IS THE RIGHT WAY TO CLEAN MY CHILD'S TEETH?

When it comes to cleaning your child's teeth, it's important to continue doing so until they develop the dexterity to brush effectively on their own, which is usually around age six or seven with adult supervision. For younger children, approaching them from behind and securing their heads can help prevent them from moving around during brushing. As they get older, you can move to a frontal approach and model proper brushing techniques for them. Consistency and persistence in establishing a routine are crucial for maintaining good oral health habits.

In terms of primary teeth, it's generally favourable to have spacing between the anterior teeth. In these cases, flossing is usually unnecessary. However, for areas where teeth are closely spaced and have contacts, such as between molars, flossing can be very helpful. Some parents may prefer to use handheld flossers, but it's important to choose a type that's gentle and easy to manipulate. Floss that glides smoothly between teeth is a good option, as this reduces the potential for the floss 'snapping' through the contact and making the child uncomfortable. It's recommended to start flossing these areas once your child begins eating solid foods, typically around the age of two and a half to three. Flossing between closely spaced teeth is crucial for maintaining good oral hygiene.

HOW CAN I ENCOURAGE MY CHILD TO BRUSH THEIR TEETH REGULARLY?

The issue of getting children to brush their teeth is a common concern among parents. It's important to establish oral hygiene habits early on in a child's life, and parents should lead by example. Demonstrating the importance of brushing regularly and making it a part of the family's routine can be very beneficial. The American Academy of Paediatrics even has a program called "Brush, Book, Bed," which encourages brushing before bedtime as a matter of routine. Children respond well to routines and modelling positive behaviour, so showing them that brushing is a positive thing can make it more likely that they'll adopt good oral hygiene habits.

As children get older, they may want to make their own choices, which can sometimes result in poor decisions. In these cases, parents can explain the benefits and consequences of their choices and encourage positive behaviour through incentives or by limiting certain privileges until they complete the necessary tasks. Overall, establishing good habits early on can make it easier to maintain good oral hygiene throughout a child's life.

HOW CAN I PREVENT TOOTH DECAY IN MY CHILD'S BABY TEETH?

There are many factors that contribute to the development of tooth decay, but some of the primary ones include the amount of bacteria in the mouth that are specifically known to cause decay. These bacteria thrive in high-acid environments, and they are often transmitted from the child's closest caregivers, particularly the mother. Therefore, it's crucial for caregivers to maintain good oral hygiene and dental health to pass along fewer harmful bacteria to the child. Maintaining a low amount of decay-causing bacteria in the mouth is essential, which can be achieved through good oral hygiene practices such as brushing and flossing regularly, as well as using fluoride toothpaste. Fluoride can help strengthen teeth and reduce the amount of harmful bacteria in the mouth.

Nutrition is also a critical factor. Consuming foods and drinks that are high in fermentable carbohydrates or simple sugars can increase the amount of time that the mouth is in a low pH state, which can weaken the tooth structure and promote the growth of decay-causing bacteria. Therefore, limiting sugar intake and consuming a balanced diet with plenty of fruits and vegetables can help maintain good oral health.

Additionally, other caregivers in the child's life should also practice good oral hygiene and have good oral health to reduce the transmission of harmful bacteria.

HOW CAN I HELP MY CHILD AVOID DENTAL INJURIES?

There are various types of dental injuries that can occur at different stages of life. While there is a broad spectrum of injuries, certain precautions can be taken to prevent them. For toddlers, childproofing the house can be very helpful in preventing falls on objects such as fireplace hearths, coffee tables, and low furniture. Covering or padding these objects can also be beneficial. As children get older and start playing sports, it's important to consider using protective gear, especially for activities with wheels that can cause impacts to the face. Helmets not only protect the head, but can contribute to the reduction in facial and oral trauma. Mouthguards can be particularly helpful in reducing oral injuries in contact sports like soccer, basketball, hockey, field hockey, wrestling, and martial arts. Pediatric dentists can assess the risk associated with certain sports and recommend suitable options for mouthguards. In the case of American football, mouthguards are typically required.

HOW CAN I HELP MY CHILD AVOID GUM DISEASE?

Good oral hygiene is crucial for maintaining healthy gums. Reducing the amount of plaque, which is a sticky substance on the teeth that can contain harmful bacteria, is key. Thorough brushing at the gum line and regular flossing are the most important steps in daily oral hygiene. Regular evaluations and cleanings with the dentist are also important to identify any problem areas and receive professional guidance on oral care. If there is a family history of significant gum disease or tooth loss, it is essential to be more diligent with oral hygiene practices, such as regular cleanings and monitoring. In some cases, genetic factors may make a person more prone to gum disease, making it crucial to work closely with the dentist to assess individual risk factors and determine the appropriate level of intervention. Tartar buildup, also known as calculus, needs to be professionally cleaned by the hygienist or dentist as it can lead to inflammation in the gum tissue known as gingivitis.

HOW CAN I HELP MY CHILD MAINTAIN GOOD ORAL HYGIENE WHILE WEARING BRACES?

First and foremost, it's important to have a discussion with the orthodontist before starting braces. Any reputable orthodontist should consider the child's hygiene history and decay risk before putting on braces. Parents should be wary of orthodontists who are eager to put braces on without discussing hygiene and decay risk. Secondly, parents should seek instruction from the orthodontist on how to maintain good oral hygiene during the braces treatment. There are also many resources available online such as social media and YouTube videos that provide information on how to properly care for braces. However, it's important to understand that it can be more challenging to keep teeth clean with braces attached, and it may take longer. It's important to embrace this and be consistent with daily maintenance.

Choosing the right professional who prioritizes hygiene and oral health and having open communication with them is key. By being diligent and consistent with at-home care and seeking guidance from the orthodontist, parents can ensure that their child's teeth are not only straight but also healthy when the braces come off.

HOW CAN I HELP MY CHILD AVOID TOOTH SENSITIVITY?

Firstly, it's important to identify the cause of sensitivity in teeth. The most common causes of sensitivity are erosion and decay. Decay can be prevented through good hygiene, proper diet low in simple sugars, adequate exposure to fluorides, and proper intake of calcium and other minerals that are essential for building and maintaining enamel.

Additionally, frequent exposure to acids is a significant problem these days, mostly due to the consumption of acidic drinks between meals, such as carbonated beverages, juice drinks, sports drinks, tea and other sweetened drinks. Sour and sticky treats are also very damaging to the enamel and can increase erosion and sensitivity.

Consuming these products in moderation and rinsing the mouth with water to dilute the acids can help reduce sensitivity. It's also crucial to work closely with a pediatric dentist to identify other possible causes of sensitivity, such as gastric reflux. In such cases, working with a physician and using alkaline rinses after acid exposures can be helpful. Overall, maintaining good hygiene, adequate fluorides, and a balanced diet are crucial for preventing sensitivity in teeth.

3.5 - DENTAL WORK

by Dr. RICHARD SIMPSON FROM USA 🏳️

WHAT ARE THE MOST COMMON DENTAL PROBLEMS IN CHILDREN?

Tooth decay is the most common chronic disease of childhood, affecting children at a rate five times higher than asthma. Despite this, it is also the most preventable disease of childhood.

WHAT CAN I DO IF MY CHILD HAS A DENTAL EMERGENCY?

If your child has a dental emergency, the first step is to have a dental home. This means having a relationship with a dentist and knowing their emergency policies, so you can get guidance on when to have your child evaluated. Many dentists offer call services, and some also offer teledentistry services that allow you to have an online evaluation with a dentist or a teledentistry company. If you don't have a dental home or are unable to access teledentistry, and your child is experiencing significant swelling or trauma, then going to an urgent care centre or the emergency room may be necessary.

However, keep in mind that these facilities will not be able to perform dentistry procedures and are therefore not the most cost-effective or desirable option. In cases where urgent care is required, these facilities may provide antibiotics to address any immediate issues, but your child will still need to be referred to a dentist for further care.

IS IT NECESSARY FOR MY CHILD TO HAVE DENTAL X-RAYS TAKEN?

X-rays are an important tool in pediatric dentistry, providing valuable information that cannot be seen by simply looking at the teeth. The American Dental Association and pediatric dentists have developed guidelines on when X-rays are necessary, which take into account factors like age, stage of development, and risk for decay. X-rays allow us to see between the teeth, where decay can often develop without visible symptoms in the mouth. Decay in primary teeth progresses much more quickly than in permanent teeth, so detecting it early can allow for more conservative treatment options. X-rays also allow for follow-up care, monitoring the progression of decay and ensuring that previous treatments have been effective.

In addition to detecting decay, X-rays can also identify other dental and bone issues, including cysts, tumours, and impactions. They can also help us count teeth and monitor the movement of permanent teeth as they develop. X-rays are also useful in cases of dental trauma, allowing us to detect changes that may not be visible to the naked eye. Overall, X-rays are an essential part of a thorough dental evaluation, providing important information that can lead to more effective treatment and better oral health outcomes. While there are risks associated with X-rays, current technology and protective procedures have greatly reduced these risks, and the benefits outweigh them in most cases. Your child's dentist can provide guidance on when X-rays are necessary and what types of X-rays are appropriate for your child's age and individual needs.

WHAT IS THE BEST WAY TO TREAT A CHILD'S CAVITIES?

When it comes to treating decay in children's teeth, several factors come into play. The first thing to consider is the extent of the decay. If it is caught early, there are conservative approaches that can be used to remineralize the affected area and stop the decay from progressing. Professional fluoride varnish treatments and super silver diamine fluoride can be effective in stopping early decay lesions in special needs children and young children. For more advanced decay, cavitated areas can be restored using a variety of materials. Modified glass ionomers and tooth-coloured composite resins are popular options, although silver amalgam is still used in some cases. For larger lesions, full-coverage restorations like stainless steel or porcelain crowns may be necessary. The choice of material depends on the dentist's skill set, the extent of the treatment needs and risks for future decay, their comfort level in treating children, and the success rates associated with each material.

In some cases, it may be possible to monitor the decay rather than treating it immediately. This approach is appropriate if the decay is not likely to progress or if it can be arrested and stabilized with conservative treatments. Your child's dentist can help you understand the best approach for your child's specific situation. Overall, the key to the successful treatment of decay in children is catching it early and using conservative approaches whenever possible. Regular dental check-ups and good oral hygiene habits are the best way to prevent decay from developing in the first place.

WHAT IS DENTAL SEALANT, AND IS IT NECESSARY FOR MY CHILD?

Dental sealant is a thin, plastic coating that is applied to the chewing surfaces of the back teeth, which are the molars and premolars. These teeth have grooves and pits that can be difficult to clean properly, making them more prone to cavities. Dental sealants fill in these grooves and pits, creating a smooth surface that is easier to clean and less likely to trap food particles and bacteria. Sealants are a preventive measure that can help protect your child's teeth from decay. They are typically recommended for children around the age of 6, when their permanent molars start to come in. The first permanent molars usually come in between the ages of 6 and 7, and the second permanent molars come in between the ages of 11 and 14.

While sealants are not necessary for every child, they can be a helpful tool in preventing cavities in children who are at higher risk for decay. Factors that can increase a child's risk of cavities include poor oral hygiene, a diet high in sugary and acidic foods and drinks, and a history of cavities. Your child's dentist can evaluate their individual risk factors and recommend sealants if they are deemed necessary. Sealants are a quick and painless procedure that can be done in just one dental visit. The sealant material is applied to the tooth surface and then cured with a special light to bond it in place. Sealants can last for several years with proper care and maintenance, but they will eventually wear down and need to be reapplied.

WHAT ARE THE BENEFITS OF ORTHODONTIC TREATMENT FOR CHILDREN?

There are several benefits to correcting misaligned teeth in children. Firstly, improving the appearance of the child's teeth can boost their self-confidence and self-esteem. Secondly, correcting misalignments can improve the function of the child's teeth. For example, open bites can make it difficult to bite into certain foods, affecting a child's ability to chew and digest properly. Thirdly, correcting misalignments can improve oral hygiene and periodontal health. Overlapping or crooked teeth can make it harder to clean the teeth properly, which can lead to gum disease and tooth decay.

IS IT OKAY FOR MY CHILD TO PLAY SPORTS WITH BRACES?

It's important to consider the added risks that come with wearing braces when participating in sports. Trauma to the mouth and brackets can cause injuries that could have been avoided with the use of a mouth guard. To ensure the child's safety, it's crucial to have a conversation with the dentist overseeing the child's braces treatment to discuss the sports they're involved in and whether they would benefit from a mouthguard. Custom or suck-down mouth guards are not suitable for patients with braces as the teeth are constantly moving.

Orthodontic sports guards are specifically designed to fit over the teeth and appliances, allowing for movement and reducing the potential for dental and oral tissue trauma, as well as the risk of concussions. Dentists providing the braces should have these available or provide instructions on how to obtain them. While they may not stay in like custom mouthguard, they are designed to be easy to breathe and speak with during sports activities. It's important to prioritize the child's safety and take necessary precautions while they're undergoing orthodontic treatment to avoid any unnecessary injuries.

WHAT ARE THE RISKS OF NOT TREATING MY CHILD'S CAVITIES?

It's important to address dental issues in children early on to prevent potential problems from becoming bigger and more costly down the road. Common issues include malocclusion, pain, and infections that can spread and cause significant facial swelling and even impact overall health. Baby teeth may not seem important since they will eventually fall out, but they have a full root and can cause infections that may damage the developing permanent teeth underneath. Self-esteem is also a factor as children can be self-conscious about obvious decay, affecting their confidence and social development. Financial concerns may also arise, but addressing dental issues earlier on with a more conservative approach is more cost-effective in the long run. Additionally, reducing active decay can decrease the risk of developing new cavities since the bacteria that cause decay can increase with more decay present.

HOW CAN I PREVENT BABY BOTTLE TOOTH DECAY IN MY CHILD?

To prevent early childhood tooth decay, it's important to first recognize that the term "baby bottle tooth decay" is outdated and not recognized in dentistry. Instead, it's referred to as early childhood caries or tooth decay. The best way to prevent it is to avoid introducing sugary drinks such as juice to children under 18-24 months and limiting their exposure to these drinks between meals and especially before bed. Water is the best option before bed as we produce less saliva at night, which is our natural defence against acid and sugar in our mouth. It's also recommended to limit the frequency of exposure to sugary drinks and avoid sippy cups that encourage frequent sips throughout the day, unless they contain only water. Drinking two to four ounces in one sitting is better than sipping the same amount throughout the day. By reducing the frequency and amount of sugary drinks and introducing healthy habits early on, we can prevent early childhood tooth decay and promote good oral health for our children.

HOW CAN I FIND A PAEDIATRIC DENTIST FOR MY CHILD?

When searching for a paediatric dentist, it's important to consider a few factors. First and foremost, ensure that the dentist is a specialist in paediatric dentistry and not just someone who treats children in a general dental practice. Additionally, look for a dentist who is board certified in their specialty. While it's not required, most paediatric dentists choose to pursue certification, which involves additional testing and continuing education. Word-of-mouth recommendations from friends, family, or other parents can be a valuable resource, as can researching the dentist's reputation and reviews online. Take the time to visit their website and learn more about their approach to caring for children's oral health. By considering these factors, you can feel confident in your choice of a paediatric dentist and trust that your child is receiving the best possible care.

HOW CAN I HELP MY CHILD MAINTAIN GOOD ORAL HYGIENE WHILE WEARING APPLIANCES?

When it comes to maintaining good oral hygiene while wearing appliances, there are a few things you can do to ensure your child's teeth and gums stay healthy. First, it's important to brush and floss regularly, ideally after every meal. This can be more challenging with braces, so consider using an interdental brush or floss threader to help reach between wires and brackets. Secondly, make sure your child avoids hard, sticky, and sugary foods that can get stuck in the appliances and increase the risk of decay. Instead, encourage them to eat a healthy and balanced diet rich in fruits, vegetables, and lean protein.

Finally, regular dental check-ups and cleanings are essential to monitor your child's progress and make any necessary adjustments to the appliances. Your orthodontist can also provide additional tips and recommendations for maintaining good oral hygiene while wearing braces or other appliances.

3.6 - FEAR/PAIN

by Dr. RICHARD SIMPSON FROM USA 🇺🇸

IS SEDATION DENTISTRY NECESSARY FOR CHILDREN?

The use of sedation in paediatric dentistry is an important part of providing quality care, especially for young children who may have extensive treatment needs or are pre-cooperative. However, the type of sedation used and whether it is safe depends on the dentist's training and experience, as well as the child's health status. Sedation carries risks, just like any other medical procedure, but the risks can be minimized when the guidelines of the American Academy of Paediatric Dentistry are followed and the dentist is adequately prepared for emergencies. It is important for parents to research their child's dentist, including their experience with sedation and their adherence to safety guidelines. In some cases, sedation may need to be done in a hospital setting for higher-risk children with medical conditions that require more intensive monitoring, or for children with more extensive and lengthy treatment needs that may not be possible to complete during a less deep sedation more commonly performed in the office such as conscious oral sedation.

HOW CAN I HELP MY CHILD COPE WITH TOOTH LOSS?

Let's discuss different scenarios of losing teeth and how to handle them. When a child is losing a tooth naturally, it's usually an exciting time for them. However, some children may feel anxious, especially if their parents have passed on their own fears or discomfort with wiggly teeth. As a dental professional, you can reassure the child that losing a tooth is a natural process of growing up and an essential part of improving their smile.

On the other hand, a traumatic loss of a tooth due to injury can be distressing for the child, especially if it's a permanent tooth. In this case, it's crucial to be empathetic and acknowledge their concerns. Show them that you understand and care about their loss. Discuss with them the various treatments available in paediatric dentistry, such as removable or fixed devices that can maintain space and restore esthetics and function, depending on their age and growth. You can also show them pictures of these options to help them feel reassured. It's essential to maintain a professional, understanding, and confident tone and language when discussing such topics with parents and children. Remember, the goal is to provide comfort and assurance while explaining different options for treatment.

HOW CAN I RELIEVE MY CHILD'S TOOTH ERUPTION PAIN?

For infants and toddlers who are teething and getting their primary teeth, it's important to be conservative in our approach. The two most common remedies that have been shown to be helpful are pressure and coolness. I advise parents to massage their child's gums or provide something safe for them to chew on like a cool teething ring or a clean, moist washcloth. However, it's not recommended to use over-the-counter numbing agents for teething, as they can be a safety issue and in rare cases may cause a disorder that reduces the ability of red blood cells to carry oxygen. It's important to note that under the age of two and a half to three, topical numbing agents should not be used. If the child is tremendously uncomfortable, I advise parents to consider giving them acetaminophen orally.

WHAT ARE THE RISKS OF USING TEETHING GELS AND CREAMS?

Teething gels and creams that contain benzocaine or lidocaine can be harmful to infants and young children. These substances can cause methemoglobinemia, a rare but serious condition that reduces the amount of oxygen carried in the bloodstream. Symptoms of methemoglobinemia can include pale or gray-coloured skin, lips, and nail beds, shortness of breath, fatigue, confusion, headache, lightheadedness, and rapid heart rate. In addition to methemoglobinemia, teething gels and creams can also cause allergic reactions, irritation, and pain in the mouth and gums. Some products may also contain sugar or other sweeteners that can contribute to tooth decay.

It is recommended that parents and caregivers avoid using teething gels and creams that contain benzocaine or lidocaine and instead try other remedies such as chilled teething rings, a clean damp washcloth to chew on, or gently massaging the baby's gums with a clean finger. If a child is experiencing significant discomfort, it is best to consult with a pediatrician or dentist for advice on safe and effective treatment options.

HOW CAN I HELP MY CHILD RECOVER AFTER A DENTAL PROCEDURE?

The level of aftercare required for a child after a dental procedure can vary depending on the type of procedure. For minor procedures such as placing a filling, there may be little to no recovery time needed. However, for more extensive procedures like multiple fillings or crowns that require tissue retraction or prepping underneath the gum tissue, over-the-counter pain medications like ibuprofen or acetaminophen may be appropriate for a couple of days. Of primary concern, especially for younger patients, is the potential for the child to self-harm, unknowingly, while numb.

Find out from the dentist or a team member if the child is numb from local anesthetic, which parts of the mouth are numb, and how long this may take before wearing off. Close monitoring by an adult caregiver after leaving the dental office is imperative to reduce the potential for oral trauma from sucking or biting by the child. Following extractions or tooth removal, post-surgical care will generally be provided to the parent or caregiver in writing and verbally. Be sure to follow the provided guidance and ensure adequate pain medication is taken regularly as instructed. It's important to follow the specific instructions given by the provider who administered any sedation, including monitoring the child and taking necessary precautions until they're fully recovered.

In addition to managing physical discomfort, it's important to provide emotional support to the child. Instead of focusing on perceived negatives, it's better to show encouragement and praise the child for their efforts. For example, instead of asking if something hurt or was difficult, you could say "you did a great job" or "I'm proud of you for handling that so well". By highlighting the positive aspects of the procedure and emphasizing the child's accomplishments, they'll be more likely to view future care in a positive light.

3.7 - MONEY

by Dr. RICHARD SIMPSON FROM USA

WHAT IS THE COST OF PAEDIATRIC DENTAL CARE?
Well, the cost of paediatric dental care can vary depending on the procedure and the extent of treatment required. Generally speaking, preventive care is less costly than treatment, and early intervention is less costly than waiting until the problem has become more severe. In terms of reimbursement and fees, paediatric dentistry may be significantly less expensive than general dentistry for certain procedures. For example, a root canal followed by a crown on a single tooth in an adult may cost more than treating several teeth in a child. However, the cost ultimately depends on the specifics of each case.

It's worth noting that prevention is key to reducing costs for dental care overall. As paediatric dentists, we aim to identify and address any issues early on to prevent more extensive treatment needs in the future. In cases where a child has extensive treatment needs due to severe tooth decay or other issues, the cost can be several thousand dollars, including dental care, medical care, and facility costs. Overall, it's important for parents to prioritize their child's dental health and work with their dentist to create a treatment plan that fits within their budget.

ARE INSURANCE PLANS COVERING CHILD DENTAL CARE?

Yes, dental care for children is covered by most dental insurance plans in the USA. The Affordable Care Act also has provisions to provide for preventive dental services. The extent of coverage may vary depending on the plan and the specific services required. It is important to check with your insurance provider to understand the details of your coverage. Additionally, children in families below certain levels of income are eligible for dental care through federal programs administered by individual states such as Medicaid and CHIP programs.

3.8 - HABITS

by Dr. RICHARD SIMPSON FROM USA 🇺🇸

IS THUMB-SUCKING HARMFUL TO MY CHILD'S TEETH?

When it comes to thumb-sucking, there are three things to consider: how often the child sucks their thumb, how long they do it, and how hard they suck. If the thumb is only in the mouth for a short time and not putting a lot of pressure on the teeth, there may not be any negative effects. However, if the child is sucking their thumb frequently and with a lot of force, it can cause problems. Research suggests that if a child sucks their thumb for less than six hours a day, it is unlikely to cause any significant harm.

Thumb sucking can affect the alignment of teeth, causing them to flare out or tip backwards. It can also cause a vertical force that affects the growth of the upper jaw and teeth. However, if the habit is stopped before permanent teeth come in, the changes can often self-correct. If thumb sucking is prolonged, it can also affect the upper arch of the mouth, causing it to become narrow. This can impact a child's ability to chew and function properly. It's important to address the thumb sucking early on to avoid long-term effects on oral health.

When it comes to breaking thumb-sucking habits, traditional methods like bad-tasting substances or covering up the thumb have not been shown to be particularly effective for young children. Most children outgrow the habit by kindergarten, before the first permanent teeth begin to erupt. It is common for the habit to decrease to 'sleepy time' before naps and bed. The key to successfully reducing or eliminating the habit is to reach an age for the child when they 'want' to stop but have trouble remembering. Then it can be a team approach and they can respond to various forms of reinforcement. There is really no need to waste energy or emotions in attempting to stop the habit at age 2 or 3. Instead, parents should focus on positive reinforcement when the child is old enough and seek advice from their paediatrician or paediatric dentist on the most effective approach for their child.

For children who suck their thumb subconsciously while sleeping, thumb guards that cannot be removed can be effective in halting the habit once the child is old enough to see this approach as a reminder and not a punishment. Parents should also identify and address any concomitant habits that contribute to thumb-sucking. If the child immediately starts digit sucking every time they hold their favorite blanket or toy, the habit may not be stopped until this object can be removed from the scenario.

One very effective method for appropriately selected cases involves operant conditioning, whereby the child receives reduction in desired rewards with each occurrence, but by reducing the habit, the reward for a set period is progressively larger. For example, something that is desirable to the child and can be broken down into measurable amounts can be selected, such as money in the form of coins, or blocks of screen time in increments of 5-10 minutes. A set amount for a reward at the end of one week is determined (ie $5 in dimes or one hour per day in extra screen time). Every time the child is seen sucking his or her thumb, they lose a coin or a set number of minutes of screen time, and they have to mark it off of a chart or remove the coin from a jar.

At the end of the week, whatever is left is theirs to keep. The first week may not result in much reward upon completion. Start fresh again for the next week, with a renewed reward awaiting them at the end of the week, depending on how many occurences there are of the habit. The loss of reward with each occurrence, with the reinforcement of more reward by reducing the habit can be very successful if the household is fully onboard and consistent. (I have to give credit here to Dr Gerald Samson, a pediatric dentist and orthodontist who performed the research and completed a masters thesis publication on this technique).

HOW CAN I PREVENT MY CHILD FROM GRINDING THEIR TEETH AT NIGHT?
When it comes to preventing teeth grinding, there are many factors to consider. While some medical conditions can contribute to teeth grinding, most children will outgrow the habit, particularly if it's nocturnal grinding during the primary dentition. In those cases, there is typically no need to stop it, as the stress on baby teeth is minimal. However, once permanent posterior teeth come in, grinding can lead to wear and TMJ symptoms. One potential cause of teeth grinding is certain types of malocclusion, where

the lower jaw is significantly set back from the upper jaw. Additionally, some children may grind their teeth due to obstructive sleep apnea, large tonsils, or other airway issues. If these issues are present, it may be helpful to see a paediatrician or an ear, nose, and throat doctor to address them. Orthodontic treatments may also help reduce grinding, although braces should not be used solely for this purpose.

In cases where teeth grinding persists, a soft night guard may be recommended to prevent wear on the teeth. It's important to work with a paediatric dentist or primary care provider to determine the best approach for each individual child. While grinding can be a concern, particularly as permanent teeth come in, most children will outgrow the habit, and there are steps parents can take to address the underlying causes of the grinding.

WHAT ARE THE DANGERS OF SHARING UTENSILS AND DRINKS WITH MY CHILD?

Tooth decay is now recognized as an infectious, transmissible disease caused by bacteria like strep mutans. These bacteria are typically not present at birth but are transmitted to children through saliva. Parents and caregivers can inadvertently pass on these microbes through activities like kissing or sharing utensils. To minimize transmission, it's important to maintain good oral hygiene and limit the exchange of saliva. For instance, avoid eating off utensils and then passing them to a child. Siblings, parents, and grandparents who are primary caregivers should also maintain good oral health to reduce the risk of transmitting harmful bacteria to children.

HOW CAN I HELP MY CHILD AVOID JAW PROBLEMS?

It's important to note that some jaw problems may be inherited and cannot be prevented. However, certain factors such as airway obstruction, habits like digit sucking or pacifier use, stress, and trauma can contribute to jaw problems. It's important to work with a paediatrician or paediatric dentist to identify these factors and address them accordingly. Coping skills, relaxation techniques, and stress management can also be helpful in managing jaw pain and dysfunction. When it comes to TMJ dysfunction, it's important to differentiate between joint pain caused by organic factors and pain caused by neuromuscular tension. Addressing habits that stress the jaw and avoiding hard or sticky foods can be helpful, and wearing a mouth guard during sports can reduce trauma to the jaw. In cases of structural problems, a proper referral to a specialist may be necessary.

HOW CAN I PREVENT DENTAL PROBLEMS IN MY CHILD WHILE THEY ARE SLEEPING?

Preventing tooth decay at night starts with limiting sugary foods and drinks before bedtime. Stick to water and ensure thorough oral hygiene before going to sleep. While nursing has many benefits, once a child starts eating solid foods, it's essential to monitor their sugar intake during the day and avoid nursing while sleeping, as it can lead to tooth decay. Thumb-sucking is a common habit among children, and if it persists at night, consider using a thumb guard with the help of a paediatrician or dentist once the child is old enough, usually at least age 5. Finally, ensure that your child is not experiencing any airway problems that could affect their quality of sleep and overall health. Good oral hygiene, a balanced diet, and regular dental visits can go a long way in maintaining healthy teeth and gums.

This is **ALPHA DENTISTRY vol. 3, PAEDIATRIC DENTISTRY FAQ**.
Welcome to the Alphas.

Dr. BAK NGUYEN

127

Dr. MARILYN SANDOR,
DDS, MS

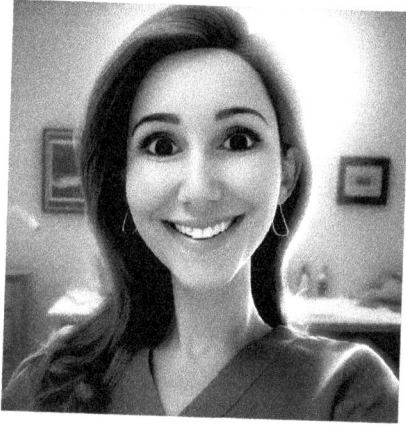

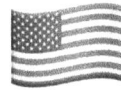

From the USA 🇺🇸, **Dr. MARILYN SANDOR**, DDS, MS, is one of Southwest Florida's favourite paediatric dentists. She is highly experienced in her field, having founded her private practice, Naples Paediatric Dentistry in the beautiful community of Naples, Florida in 2001. Dr. Sandor is a successful business owner and an active member of her community. She is committed to educating her young patients on the importance of oral health and enjoys teaching children how to have healthy smiles for a lifetime. Dr. Sandor's paediatric-focused invention, Zooby prophy angles, inspired a full line of creative new products by Young Innovations, which have been bringing joy to dental patients around the world for over a decade. She is the founder and CEO of the GoodCheckup Corporation, a new software company that provides easily accessible and equitable platforms for dentists to expand their reach via a mobile-to-mobile, patent-pending, teledentistry solution. GoodCheckup's flagship products, GoodCheckup Patient and GoodCheckup Doctor are the first Cloud-based, comprehensive smartphone teledentistry applications created by a paediatric dentist specifically for paediatric dentistry.

Dr. Marilyn Sandor and I were introduced by Dr. Paul Dominique. Even if we just met, Dr. Sandor has been a force of nature within the Alphas, co-signing 2 books, including this one, and being a very active Alpha recruiting international experts for the other teams.

An experienced practitioner herself, kind and dedicated, Marilyn is also an entrepreneur with the vision to change the landscape of our profession. She is deploying a new concept for practicing paediatric dentistry combining prevention, technology and human touch.

I feel blessed to exchange and collaborate with Alphas like Dr. Sandor. I said once before in an international interview: "They are not my Alphas, they are Alphas." Well, Marilyn is the testament to that. She is a force of nature and an Alpha, I just had the fortune to be introduced to her. Now, together, as Alphas, let's see what we can achieve. Please join me in welcoming Dr. Marilyn Sandor into the Alphas.

This is **ALPHA DENTISTRY vol. 3, PAEDIATRIC DENTISTRY FAQ**. Welcome to the Alphas.

Dr. BAK NGUYEN

CHAPTER 4

"PAEDIATRIC DENTISTRY"

by Dr. MARILYN SANDOR

FROM USA 🇺🇸

4.1 - DEFINITIONS

by Dr. MARILYN SANDOR FROM USA

WHAT IS THE BEST TYPE OF TOOTHBRUSH FOR MY CHILD?

When it comes to choosing a toothbrush for a child, the most important factor is finding one that they will use consistently. A toothbrush with soft or extra-soft bristles is ideal for children. However, the most crucial aspect is how effectively the toothbrush removes plaque. Acheiving effective plaque removal can be done with either a manual toothbrush or an electric toothbrush. Though an electric toothbrush by design quickly disrupts and dislodges plaque buildup by motorized movement, a manual toothbrush can also be effective using good technique. When selecting either an electric or manual toothbrush, consider the child user's age, personality and level of dexterity.

Age of the user is relevant in selecting the physical size and handle design of a toothbrush. A size-appropriate brush head will achieve better results. If the head of the toothbrush is sized to contact one or two teeth at a time, one can achieve better plaque removal. Personality of the child user is important from a motivational standpoint. Colors and characters that the child enjoys can increase a child's willingness to engage in tooth brushing. The manual dexterity of the child must also be considered, as brushing efficacy has a direct relationship. Select a toothbrush with a handle that is suited proportionately for the user. Also consider whether the vibration of the electric toothbrush itself may make the brush more difficult to grasp. With these concepts in mind, you will be well equipped to make the best selection for your child. Remember to assist your child with brushing and keep a positive attitude.

WHAT IS THE ROLE OF FLUORIDE IN PREVENTING CAVITIES?

When it comes to fluoride, it's important to understand its role in protecting our teeth. Fluoride is a naturally occurring element that can help strengthen the enamel and make it more resistant to acid attacks from bacteria and acidic foods. This is particularly important for children, whose teeth are still developing and more vulnerable to decay.

There are different ways to apply fluoride, such as toothpaste, fluoride varnish, and sealants. Each method has its own benefits and limitations. Toothpaste is the most common and convenient way to apply fluoride, but it's important to use it in moderation and supervise young children so they do not eat the toothpaste or swallow large quantities. Fluoride varnish offers a more concentrated form of fluoride that is applied by a dental professional and can provide longer-lasting protection. Sealants can also offer slow release fluoride. Glass ionomer sealants are a material which contains fluoride and can be applied to the chewing surfaces of the back teeth to prevent bacteria from settling in the grooves.

It's important to note that fluoride alone cannot prevent cavities. Good oral hygiene practices, such as brushing twice a day, flossing, and regular dental check-ups, are also crucial in maintaining a healthy smile. So, when it comes to fluoride, it's all about finding the right balance and using it as part of a comprehensive oral care routine.

WHAT IS THE DIFFERENCE BETWEEN A PAEDIATRIC DENTIST AND A GENERAL DENTIST?

The comparison between a paediatric dentist and a family dentist is similar to the difference between a paediatrician and a general practitioner. A paediatric dentist is focused on children's oral health from birth to young adulthood, and they have a deep understanding of their growth and development during these years. They are specialized in the how and why of maintaining children's teeth and helping parents understand that a healthy dentition will aid in proper growth and development, including facial proportions. In contrast, a general dentist may have some familiarity with childhood dentistry, but it is most often not their primary focus. A paediatric dentist has undergone additional training in formal residency programs that give them more knowledge and experience in this specific field. They work closely with medical colleagues and are better equipped to guide parents through this crucial and sensitive period of their child's life.

WHAT ARE THE MOST COMMON ORTHODONTIC PROBLEMS IN CHILDREN?

When it comes to common orthodontic problems, the most frequent issue is crowding. However, there are other orthodontic problems that may arise due to premature loss of primary teeth or failure to identify a problem early on. For example, ectopically erupting canines or first molars can cause malocclusion if left untreated. A paediatric dentist can check for these issues during routine dental exams and guide parents on when to seek orthodontic treatment.

While a paediatric dentist may not perform orthodontic procedures, they will refer patients to an orthodontist if necessary. During routine dental exams, a paediatric dentist will check the child's bite alignment and dental development to determine if orthodontic treatment is necessary. They will also monitor the child's dental health over time and provide guidance on when it is appropriate to seek an orthodontic evaluation.

HOW CAN I TELL IF MY CHILD NEEDS ORTHODONTIC TREATMENT?

There are several signs that may indicate that your child needs orthodontic treatment. These include crowded or crooked teeth, teeth that are not aligned properly, difficulty biting or chewing, early or late loss of baby teeth. Thumb sucking or other oral habits may affect a child's bite, resulting in the need for orthodontic treatment. Jaw clicking or popping, speech difficulties or problems with pronunciation also may be an indication of orthodontic needs. If you notice any of these signs, it may be a good idea to consult with a pediatric dentist or an orthodontist for an evaluation to determine if your child needs orthodontic treatment.

WHAT ARE THE BENEFITS OF DENTAL SEALANTS FOR CHILDREN?

Fluoride acts as a sunscreen, while dental sealants function like a sun shirt. Sealants are applied as a physical barrier to the chewing surfaces of back teeth, sealing off crevices and preventing food particles from getting trapped in the creases and causing cavities. The application of a sealant reduces the chance for developing cavities in those areas. Sealants can last anywhere from three to five years, with some lasting up to ten years, depending on wear and tear and the depth of the crevices.

When it comes to cost, sealants are much more affordable, typically costing one-third to one-quarter the price of a filling. Preventing cavities with sealants is definitely worth it because not only is it more affordable, but it also helps avoid drilling into the tooth and adding a synthetic material which may need to be replaced later on.

As for applying sealants to baby teeth, it is a selective process for me. Before the development of self-etching adhesives, applying sealants to young children could be a struggle and may frighten them due to the water rinsing and noise-producing suction equipment involved during the application process. I would only recommend it on primary teeth if there are specific needs, such as deep crevices or hypo-mineralized teeth. For permanent teeth, if there is a crevice, in general, it is best to apply a sealant to prevent cavities.

4.2 - PREVENTION

by Dr. MARILYN SANDOR FROM USA 🇺🇸

HOW CAN I PREPARE MY CHILD FOR THEIR FIRST DENTAL VISIT?

There are a few ways to approach preparing children for their first dental visit, depending on the parents' perception of dentistry and their child's anxiety levels. For some parents, it may be best to keep the explanation simple and surface-level, sharing with the child that the dentist will take care of their teeth to make the teeth happy and shiny. This approach can help the child view the visit as a positive experience and engage them in learning about self-care for the future.

In terms of when the first dental visit should occur, the American Academy of Paediatric Dentistry recommends that it should be by the child's first tooth or first birthday. Starting early with preventative care is crucial for a lifetime of good oral health, and pediatric dentists can provide guidance and education for parents even before the baby is born. Pediatric dentists often counsel parents on how to avoid early childhood cavities, which is often caused by putting a child to bed with a bottle. Further, dental professionals can encourage parents to offer children water or milk only as their beverages of choice, which will greatly lessen the risks for developing tooth decay, often associated with the consumption of juices and sweetened drinks.

HOW CAN I HELP MY CHILD OVERCOME THEIR FEAR OF THE DENTIST?

To address a child's fear of the dentist, it's important to first understand why they are fearful. Did they have a bad experience in the past or hear something negative from someone else? Once you have identified the source of their fear, you can take steps to address it. One strategy is to use positive language when discussing the dental visit. Emphasize that the dentist is there to help keep their teeth healthy and strong and that the visit will be a pleasant one. You can also allow the child to hold a mouth mirror to familiarize with them a dental instrument.

Another approach is to use desensitization techniques, such as progressive exposure to the dental office and equipment. This can help the child become more comfortable and familiar with the environment and reduce their anxiety. Above all, it's important to approach the child's fears with compassion and understanding. Acknowledge their feelings and validate their concerns. By building trust and making the experience as positive and comfortable as possible, you can help alleviate their fears and make the dental visit a successful one.

HOW CAN I PREPARE MY CHILD FOR A DENTAL PROCEDURE?

When it comes to preparing your child for a dental procedure, it's important to ease any fears or anxiety they may have. One effective way to do this is by focusing on a pleasant part of the experience, such being able to listen to music or watch a movie during the procedure. If the patient is young and not yet able to fully understand the purpose of the visit and the long term gain of the procedure, using nitrous oxide, can help them through a dental procedure, in that not only can aid with anxiety and pain, in can be an enjoyable distraction from the procedure itself. For example, you can tell them that they'll be wearing a cool mask on their nose and they will feel like they're floating on a cloud. Reassure them that the procedure is very normal and that the dentist knows exactly what they're doing. If you want to, you can also promise them a fun activity or treat afterwards as a reward. The most important thing is to make sure they feel comfortable and confident going into the procedure.

IS IT OKAY FOR CHILDREN TO CONSUME SUGARY FOODS AND DRINKS?

Let me start by saying that sugar can be a problem, but it's not always the problem. The way you consume it and the types of sugar you consume are also important factors to consider. When counseling parents, it's important to avoid being too strict, as it can be overwhelming and it may not be sustainable in the long run. Understanding family dynamics and social factors is an important part of developing a plan for a diet that is less likely to cause cavities. I suggest starting with small modifications to their diet, such as focusing on drinks first. Encourage children to drink lots of water and to select water or milk as their primary beverage. From there, we can look at the types of sugary foods they are consuming and find ways to modify their diet to make it better. For example, if it is a processed food, it may be more cariogenic because it may have a greater tendency to cling to the teeth, whereas a homemade cookie may be easier to brush off. Ultimately, we need to dig deeper into the specific circumstances and find a solution that works best for each individual family.

When discussing diet with parents, it's important to consider the specific types of food and drinks consumed, rather than simply focusing on sugar content. For example, a snack like processed goldfish crackers with apple juice could be more concerning than a treat like a frosted donut with milk because the sticky texture of the crackers and juice can create a very difficult to remove plaque residue. On the other hand, the donut with milk, a much less sticky and non acidic drink, can be easily brushed away. It's important to have a conversation with parents about specific foods and drinks, and work together to make reasonable modifications to promote good oral health.

CAN MY CHILD STILL ENJOY SWEET TREATS WHILE MAINTAINING GOOD ORAL HYGIENE?
It's difficult to give a blanket answer to this question as it depends on what kind of sweet treats we're talking about. Generally, sweets that can be easily brushed off

your teeth, such as chocolates, can be enjoyed as long as you maintain good oral hygiene. During holidays, such as Halloween in the USA, it is common to treat children with candy. I advise parents that from a dental health perspective, not to give their children the candies that have colours. These colored, generally hard or sticky candies, linger in their mouth for a long time, giving the sugar and the bacteria that digest that sugar, plenty of time to do damage. As for chocolate, it's less acidic and destructive to the teeth due to its milk content. Home-baked cupcakes, cakes, or pies can also be enjoyed as long as you can clean them off your teeth. It's important to remember to maintain good oral hygiene, though.

Regarding pH levels, I believe that neutral is the best for maintaining dental health. Drinking only water with your meals is much better for your teeth than brushing frequently but still consuming juices or other acidic drinks. Lemon in water can also decalcify teeth over time, so it's best to be cautious.

In conclusion, it's not a joke to say that chocolate can be okay for your teeth as long as you brush it off. Dark chocolate, for example, has flavonoids that are actually good for your teeth. However, it's important to remember that everything should be consumed in moderation and that maintaining good oral hygiene is key.

HOW CAN I ENSURE MY CHILD IS RECEIVING ADEQUATE NUTRITION FOR HEALTHY TEETH?
To promote optimal dental health for children, it's essential to be mindful of what they drink. Water and milk are the best options, as sugary drinks can lead to

cavities. Making small changes, like substituting one sugary drink for water each day, can make a big difference over time. However, it's important to remember that every family is unique and what works for one may not work for another.

In addition to monitoring beverage consumption, it's important to be aware of potential sources of decay-causing bacteria. Caretakers, including nannies and daycare providers, should be screened for healthy teeth and recent dental exams to prevent the transmission of bacteria by sharing utensils or blowing on food to cool it, when feeding a young child. Parents should also take a close look at their child's diet; reducing processed foods and sticky snacks will help lower the risk of tooth decay.

Lastly, I recommend avoiding gummy vitamins and gummy candies. I feel that the residue left on the teeth can contribute to cavities. It's worth noting that brushing teeth and physically removing food debris are also essential steps in preventing cavities. By taking these proactive measures, parents can help their children maintain optimal dental health.

HOW CAN I ENSURE MY CHILD IS GETTING ENOUGH FLUORIDE?

I think it's important to consider each individual case and assess whether the child is at risk for cavities or not. If the child is at low risk and has access to fluoridated water, this is adequte and a conservative approach is appropriate. However, if the child is at high risk for cavities, then fluoride treatments may be recommended. It is also important to consider the child's diet and whether any modifications can be made to reduce the risk of cavities. In some cases, higher fluoride content toothpaste or other fluoride treatments may be advised. If a child's teeth have enamel defects, such as those caused by inadequae oral hygiene causing decalcification or from heredetary defects. Ultimately, it's about finding the right balance and providing individualized care based on each child's unique needs.

HOW CAN I PREVENT ORTHODONTIC PROBLEMS IN MY CHILD?

To prevent your child from experiencing orthodontic problems, the best thing you can do is to keep their primary teeth in good health. These teeth act as placeholders for the permanent teeth, so if a baby tooth falls out prematurely, it can result in shifting and lead to orthodontic problems down the road. It's important to keep up with regular dental check-ups and catch any issues early on.

When it comes to orthodontic treatment, it's best to seek advice as early as possible, ideally when the child is around 8 years old or even sooner. It's important to identify any potential problems early on and address them before they become more serious. Seeking advice from an orthodontist at a young age can also help guide the growth and development of the child's teeth and jaws, potentially avoiding the need for more extensive treatment.

4.3 - TIME

by Dr. MARILYN SANDOR FROM USA

WHAT IS THE BEST AGE FOR A CHILD TO START SEEING A DENTIST?

The best age for a child to start seeing a dentist is around the age of one, or when their first tooth erupts, whichever comes first. This is because early dental visits can help parents learn how to properly care for their child's teeth and gums and detect any potential dental problems from the start. Additionally, regular dental visits can establish a positive relationship between the child and the dentist, helping to alleviate fear and anxiety surrounding dental visits in the future.

HOW OFTEN SHOULD MY CHILD SEE A DENTIST?

When it comes to scheduling dental checkups for children, it depends on their individual needs, but generally, having an examination every six months is recommended. Children are continuously growing and developing; changes occur rapidly and a six-month interval allows a dentist to monitor closely and address specific care needs promptly.

WHAT IS THE BEST AGE FOR A CHILD TO GET ORTHODONTIC TREATMENT?

It is advisable for children to undergo an orthodontic screening around the age of eight. After a child changes over their baby incisors, which are the upper and lower four front teeth, there is usually a span of one to two years, before the remaining primary teeth change over. Generally speaking, it is between this time that an orthodontic screening is recommended. The purpose of an orthodontic consultation is to aid in identifying common orthodontic problems such as overcrowding, misaligned teeth, and bite issues. There will be an evaluation of the child's dental and facial development and guidance will be given on whether orthodontic treatment is necessary. Early intervention can save parents time and money and prevent future dental issues.

Regarding the best age to have an evaluation for possible orthodontic treatment, an initial screening around age eight is often recommended since the child's jaw has usually developed enough to assess any potential orthodontic issues. However, treatment may begin earlier if a child is experiencing problems with the baby teeth falling out or if a panoramic X-ray shows that early intervention is necessary. The goal is to recognize and address any orthodontic needs at the appropriate time to ensure optimal oral health and development for children.

WHAT ARE THE SIGNS OF TEETH ERUPTION IN A CHILD?
When a baby starts teething, they may show typical signs such as increased drooling and a desire to chew or gnaw on things. Some babies may also become cranky during this time, but not all experience pain or fever. It can vary even within the same family, with some children having more difficulty than others. If a baby is experiencing pain or discomfort, there are options such as giving them a cool teething ring to chew. Acetaminophen for children may also be recommended if the pain is significant and is causing distress.

4.4 - MAINTENANCE

by Dr. MARILYN SANDOR FROM USA

WHAT IS THE RIGHT WAY TO CLEAN MY CHILD'S TEETH?

To properly clean a child's teeth, it's recommended to brush gently with small back and forth motions, aiming for where the gum and tooth come together. This helps remove plaque and prevent gum disease. As for how long a child should brush their teeth, the standard recommendation is two minutes, but it's more important to focus on thoroughness rather than a specific time. Make sure to brush all surfaces, including the top, inside, and chewing surfaces of the teeth. If the child has a hard time brushing for two minutes, using a timer or an app can help. Ultimately, the goal is to ensure the child's teeth are thoroughly cleaned to promote good oral health.

HOW CAN I ENCOURAGE MY CHILD TO BRUSH THEIR TEETH REGULARLY?

Encouraging children to brush their teeth regularly can be challenging, but there are a few strategies you can try. Firstly, make brushing a fun activity by letting them choose their own toothbrush and toothpaste with their favourite character or flavour. You can also make a game out of brushing by setting a timer for two minutes and challenging your child to brush for the entire time. Additionally, create a routine by setting a specific time for brushing each morning and night, and make sure to lead by example by brushing your own teeth alongside your child. Praising and rewarding your child for brushing well can also motivate them to continue the habit. Finally, educate them about the importance of brushing to maintaining healthy teeth and a bright smile. With patience and consistency, you can help your child develop good oral hygiene habits that will last a lifetime.

HOW CAN I PREVENT TOOTH DECAY IN MY CHILD'S BABY TEETH?

To help prevent tooth decay in your child's baby teeth, it is good practice to brush your child's teeth twice a day with a pea-sized amount of fluoridated toothpaste and if warranted, where teeth are tightly aligned, floss daily. Encourage your child to eat a balanced diet and limit sugary and acidic foods and avoid sweetened drinks, as these can erode tooth enamel and contribute to decay. Consider having dental sealants applied to your child's molars, which can provide an extra layer of protection against decay. Regular dental check-ups are also an important part of a preventive care plan. Educatating your child, starting at a young age, about the importance of good oral hygiene and the consequences of poor dental health is also very important. By taking these steps, you can help your child maintain a healthy and bright smile.

HOW CAN I PREVENT MY CHILD FROM DEVELOPING DENTAL ANXIETY?

Starting dental visits at a young age can help establish a positive experience and build trust with the dentist. Parents can play a role in promoting dental care as a self-care activity, similar to other aspects of hygiene and health. It's important to avoid using fear tactics or making threats related to dental visits, as this can lead to dental anxiety. If a child has a strong gag reflex or discomfort with a procedure, forcing them can exacerbate their anxiety. Instead, dentists should approach treatment with sensitivity and guide the child to make their own decisions. By taking a positive and nuanced approach to dental care, parents and dentists can help establish a foundation for good dental health throughout a child's life.

HOW CAN I HELP MY CHILD AVOID DENTAL INJURIES?

To prevent dental injuries, it's important to take proactive measures. Encouraging the use of mouthguards during contact sports or activities is one effective way to protect teeth from impact. Parents should also prioritize teaching their children proper brushing and flossing techniques to prevent gum disease and tooth decay, which can lead to other dental issues down the line. It's important to avoid chewing on hard objects like ice or popcorn kernels, which can cause tooth fractures or breakages. Regular dental check-ups are essential to catching potential issues early on and preventing them from becoming more serious.

In addition to these preventative measures, it's important for parents to be aware of potential tripping hazards in the home such as rugs that aren't fixed and to supervise toddlers in the bathtub or pool. Children are at risk of hitting their teeth on the edge of the bathtub or pool, leading to serious dental injuries. To prevent dangerous falls, parents should also be mindful when drying a child after a bath and avoid wrapping them tightly in a towel without leavning their arms free. By being mindful of these potential hazards, parents can help protect their child's dental health and overall safety.

Living in Florida, we often see dental injuries occur around pools and during sports. To prevent these types of injuries, it's best to avoid smiling or keeping your lips apart when approaching the edge of a pool or playing sports. This can protect your teeth from accidental hits or impacts. As a dentist, I recommend these precautions to my patients to help keep their smiles healthy and injury-free.

HOW CAN I HELP MY CHILD AVOID GUM DISEASE?

Gum disease, which can progress to gingivitis, is often caused by plaque buildup along the gum line. To prevent this, it's important to drink plenty of water to dilute the plaque and brush regularly with a soft or extra-soft brush, focusing on the gum line. Imagine it's like finger painting and you're trying to clean the paint around your cuticles - that's where you want to brush to remove plaque buildup. Flossing can also be helpful to remove larger debris, but the need for flossing depends on the alignment of teeth. If a child's teeth are widely spaced, brushing alone may be sufficient.

As for when to start flossing, it depends on the child's teeth. If the teeth are tightly spaced, parents can use disposable flossers to gently clean between teeth as early as a year and a half. For children with widely spaced teeth, brushing alone may be sufficient until around the age of five. It's always a good idea to consult with a paediatric dentist to determine the best dental care practices for your child. Additionally, regular dental check-ups can help catch and prevent gum disease and other dental issues.

HOW CAN I HELP MY CHILD MAINTAIN GOOD ORAL HYGIENE WHILE WEARING BRACES?

To maintain good oral health while wearing braces, it's important to take extra care to prevent the buildup of plaque and food particles around the brackets. This can be done by drinking plenty of water to rinse your mouth and teeth, especially after eating. When brushing, it's important to focus on the gum line above the brackets on the top teeth and below the brackets on the bottom teeth. Flossing can be challenging with braces, but there are toothbrushes on the market, like the Waterpik, that can help jet water through and under the wire to remove debris. Aim for water debris removal and targeting the gum line above and below the brackets. By following these tips, those with braces can maintain good oral health and prevent gingivitis.

HOW CAN I HELP MY CHILD AVOID TOOTH SENSITIVITY?

To address tooth sensitivity, it's important to first identify the root cause of the issue. Tooth sensitivity can occur due to various reasons such as physical injury, cavities, teething, the eruption of other teeth, poorly mineralized enamel, or even the growth of wisdom teeth. It can also occur after a dental restoration procedure. Therefore, it's crucial to determine the underlying cause of sensitivity before treatment can be recommended.

To avoid tooth sensitivity, it's essential to practice good oral hygiene and prevent cavities. Using toothpaste specifically designed to address sensitivity can also help, such as those containing amorphous calcium. Additionally, maintaining a healthy diet and avoiding acidic or sugary foods can help prevent sensitivity and tooth decay.

Overall, identifying the source of tooth sensitivity and practicing good oral hygiene can help prevent and address sensitivity issues. It's essential to visit a dentist for regular check-ups to ensure any potential issues are caught early and treated promptly.

4.5 - DENTAL WORK

by Dr. MARILYN SANDOR FROM USA 🇺🇸

WHAT ARE THE MOST COMMON DENTAL PROBLEMS IN CHILDREN?

The most common dental problems in children include tooth decay, also known as cavities, gum disease, also known as gingivitis and periodontitis, tooth sensitivity, and dental injuries. These can be caused by a variety of factors such as poor oral hygiene, a diet high in sugary or acidic foods and drinks, not wearing a mouthguard during sports, and accidents or trauma to the mouth. It's important for parents to encourage good oral hygiene habits, regular dental check-ups, and taking preventative measures to avoid dental injuries. Additionally, identifying and addressing dental problems early on can help prevent them from becoming more serious and requiring more extensive treatment.

WHAT CAN I DO IF MY CHILD HAS A DENTAL EMERGENCY?

Patients find it very helpful to schedule an emergency telehealth visit for guideance. In the case of a dental emergency, it is important to take immediate action. If a baby tooth has been knocked out, do not to try to put it back in. However, if it's a permanent tooth, you should try to reinsert it as soon as possible, being careful to touch only the crown of the tooth and not the root. Then, it's important to get to a dentist as soon as possible.

In terms of seeking medical help, a telehealth consult with a pediatric dentist can be very useful in identifying the problem and determining the best course of action. This can save you a lot of time and hassle compared to waiting in an emergency room where there may not be a dentist available. Some hospitals may not have dental professionals on staff, so it's important to be aware of your options and seek out the appropriate medical care.

IS IT NECESSARY FOR MY CHILD TO HAVE DENTAL X-RAYS TAKEN?
It's important to consider each child's individual situation when determining whether or not they need dental x-rays. For very young children x-rays may not be advised or may be difficult to take, due to the coopration level of the child. There are many reasons for recommending x-rays, some of which may be to evaluate growth and development, to screen for pathology, or to monitor a patient who is at high risk for decay. However, it's important for pediatric dentists to be judicious in prescribing x-rays and to consider the child's comfort and safety. Some children may have a strong gag reflex or feel fearful during the process of taking x-rays.

WHAT IS THE BEST WAY TO TREAT A CHILD'S CAVITIES?
It's important to catch cavities early and address them promptly with appropriate fillings. It's also important to maintain good oral hygiene habits to prevent cavities

from forming in the first place or recurring. Remineralization can be effective in treating early-stage cavities, when the decay is only in the outer layer of the enamel, but more advanced cavities will require more extensive treatment. The goal should always be to treat the cavity as minimally as possible, while ensuring that it is thorough and comfortable for the child. Overall, the best way to treat cavities in children is through a combination of preventive measures, early detection, and appropriate treatment.

WHAT IS DENTAL SEALANT, AND IS IT NECESSARY FOR MY CHILD?
Sealants are not recommended for every child and whether or not they are necessary depends on the individual child's tooth shape. If a child has deep crevices in their teeth, sealants may be a good idea to help prevent cavities. However, if a child does not have deep grooves and does not have a history of dental cavities, then sealants may not be necessary. It is important to note that poorly applied sealants can potentially cause more harm than good, so it is important to ensure that sealants are applied correctly and not leaking underneath. Sealants are technique sensitive and should be applied to a clean tooth surface. It is important to be cautious about where and how sealants are applied.

WHAT ARE THE BENEFITS OF ORTHODONTIC TREATMENT FOR CHILDREN?
To address the question of the benefits of orthodontic treatment for children, there are several reasons why it may be recommended. In cases of more severe malocclusion, orthodontic treatment can improve a child's ability to chew and eat properly, which is important for their overall nutrition and health.

Additionally, if a child has misaligned teeth or a malocclusion that affects their speech, orthodontic treatment can help improve their speech and communication skills. Lastly, many children and parents seek orthodontic treatment for aesthetic reasons, as straighter teeth can improve a child's self-esteem and confidence.

IS IT OKAY FOR MY CHILD TO PLAY SPORTS WITH BRACES?
In contact sports, it's highly recommended to wear a custom-made mouthguard that fits over the braces. This can help prevent damage to the teeth and braces in case of any impact or injury. It's important to consult with your orthodontist for recommendations on the best type of mouthguard to use for your specific situation.

WHAT ARE THE RISKS OF NOT TREATING MY CHILD'S CAVITIES?
Neglecting dental problems can lead to serious consequences such as pain, infection, swelling, hospitalization, and in rare cases, death. Decay that is left untreated can spread to the pulp and cause infection, which can spread to the gums and bone. This can cause swelling, dangerous airway obstruction, cellulitis, hospitalization and even death. It is important to address dental problems in a timely manner to avoid serious consequences.

HOW CAN I PREVENT BABY BOTTLE TOOTH DECAY IN MY CHILD?
To prevent baby bottle tooth decay, the best approach is to avoid putting the baby to bed with a bottle. It is recommended to follow a proper weaning regimen and wean the baby from the bottle or nursing at night by the age of one to prevent tooth decay.

HOW CAN I FIND A PAEDIATRIC DENTIST FOR MY CHILD?

There are several ways to find a good paediatric dentist for your child. One common way is to ask for recommendations from friends and family. Another option is to visit the website of the Academy of Paediatric Dentistry, which provides a list of recommended paediatric dentists in your area. With the availability of telehealth, virtual consultations with paediatric dentists can also be a great way to familiarize your child with the dentist before their first visit. This can help reduce anxiety and build a rapport with the dentist before meeting in person.

HOW CAN I HELP MY CHILD MAINTAIN GOOD ORAL HYGIENE WHILE WEARING APPLIANCES?

To maintain good oral hygiene with orthodontic appliances, it's important to remove removable appliances before brushing and cleaning your teeth. Drinking water and milk, or almond milk for those with allergies, can help prevent food from clinging to the appliances. In addition to good brushing habits, utilizing newer brushing tools with a built-in water flosser can also be beneficial for maintaining oral hygiene.

4.6 - FEAR/PAIN

by Dr. MARILYN SANDOR FROM USA 🇺🇸

IS SEDATION DENTISTRY NECESSARY FOR CHILDREN?

Let me start by saying that sedation should not be used for all children. There are various types of sedation dentistry, which differ by the medications used and the means they are administered. There are medical considerations for each type and sedation should be recommended based upon the patient's needs and the patient's health and abilty to cooperate with dental care. For only those children who cannot tolerate dental care otherwise, sedation dentistry offers a means to receive necessary dental care with higher saftey.

Nitrous oxide is a common analgesic used in dentistry, which can help reduce a patient's perception of unpleasant stimuli during the procedure. This is a safe and pleasant adjunct to introduce a young patient to receiving dental surgical care while awake. I feel that if care can be administered in the most gentle manner possible at a young age, the patient will likely become more tolerant and less fearful in their later years. This is why it's crucial to be comforting during a child's early years to help prevent the development of deep-seated dental anxiety which may affect them for the rest of their lives.

Sedation dentistry does, however, carry risks; the type of sedation used and the person administering are crucial. It's best to work with board-certified paediatric anesthesiologists to reduce the risks of over-sedation or choking, which could lead to unconsciousness or even death. It's important to be cautious and well-trained when using sedation dentistry to ensure all proper safeguards are in place.

HOW CAN I HELP MY CHILD COPE WITH TOOTH LOSS?
When a child loses a baby tooth naturally, it's important to reassure them that it's a normal part of growing up

and that a new, permanent tooth will replace it. You can use stories or analogies to help them understand this process, such as comparing it to getting new shoes or clothes that fit better. If a baby tooth is knocked out, you can reassure them, for example with concepts, such as the Tooth Fairy, emphasizing that a replacement tooth is already in the works.

However, if a permanent tooth is lost, it can be a traumatic experience for a child. It's important to remain calm and reassuring, letting them know that dental professionals have the technology and expertise to make things better. Remember to use positive language and avoid alarmist language that could easily increase anxiety.

HOW CAN I RELIEVE MY CHILD'S TOOTH ERUPTION PAIN?

While some people may use herbal supplements like arnica, I would recommend talking to a paediatrician before using them, especially for very young children. However, providing something for the child to chew on can be helpful in relieving teething discomfort. Teething rings that can be cooled in the refrigerator can provide some relief, and some children may also find chewing on an extra soft toothbrush helpful, particularly the plastic on the back. Ultimately, finding what works best for your child may involve some trial and error, but the goal is to provide comfort and relief during this stage of development.

WHAT ARE THE RISKS OF USING TEETHING GELS AND CREAMS?

While topical gels and creams can provide temporary relief for teething pain, they may not address the underlying cause of the pain, which is usually from the pressure of the new tooth from within. Additionally, some products may contain anesthetics that can be harmful if overused. It's important to be cautious and follow the instructions carefully if using these products. If a caregiver wishes to use organic medicaments, it's important to research and consult with a healthcare professional before using them as well. Ultimately, it's important to keep in mind that teething is a natural process and some discomfort is normal. Using a cool teething ring or extra soft toothbrush can also provide relief without the potential risks of topical products.

HOW CAN I HELP MY CHILD RECOVER AFTER A DENTAL PROCEDURE?

After a dental procedure, it's important to rest and avoid strenuous activities. If a child has received local anesthetic, it is prudent to minimize the risks for self-injury after a dental procedure. Actions, such as chewing can place a child at risk of biting their lip or tongue. To decrease that risk, if a child is hungry after their dental visit, it is best to offer only soft foods that are cool or at room temperature like yogurt.

This can be helpful to make them feel better. Ensure that they drink plenty of water and avoid talking too much, which could also lead to accidentally biting their own tongue or lips. If the child is not allergic to anelgesics, acetaminophen or ibuprofen can be helpful to decrease the risk of post-treatment paid. These medications should be taken with food, to decrease risk of stomach upset.

4.7 - MONEY

by Dr. MARILYN SANDOR FROM USA

WHAT IS THE COST OF PAEDIATRIC DENTAL CARE?

Dental care for children may be less expensive than that for adults, as children typically require less extensive treatment and may not have as many preexisting conditions. Factors such as the location of the dental practice and the type of filling material used may also affect the cost. It is important to consult with a dentist or dental insurance provider for more specific information on costs.

ARE THOSE COVERED BY THE GOVERNMENT?

While there are some government dental coverages in the US that provide for children's dental care, it is important to note that not everyone qualifies for these programs, particularly those who are over a certain income threshold.

ARE INSURANCE COVERING CHILD DENTAL CARE?

While dental insurance does cover many dental procedures, there are certain aspects that are not covered. For instance, most insurances do not cover anesthesia or other comfort measures like nitrous oxide. This can put paediatric dentists in a difficult position, especially when some parents do not understand the purpose of providing more comprehensive measures to provide comfort for their child or why anxiety reducing approaches are beneficial for long term dental compliance. While dental insurance can be helpful, there are still gaps in coverage.

4.8 - HABITS

by Dr. MARILYN SANDOR FROM USA 🇺🇸

IS THUMB-SUCKING HARMFUL TO MY CHILD'S TEETH?

It's important to approach thumb-sucking habits in a personalized way since every child is different and their habits can vary. Asking specific questions about the child's habits is crucial to determine the potential risks and make a tailored treatment plan. For instance, if a child sucks their thumb only at night, it's important to assess if it remains in their mouth all night or if it falls out after they fall asleep. If it falls out, it may not harm their teeth, but if it stays in, it could lead to malocclusions and other issues. Therefore, it's essential to examine each child's habits closely before recommending a course of action.

When addressing habits like thumb sucking, it's important to consider the frequency and timing of the habit. If the habit is causing the teeth to shift or the child's bite to become misaligned, it may be better to discourage or stop the habit before the permanent teeth erupt. This is because when the permanent teeth erupt, if the habit still persists, it can lead to more challenging orthodontic corrections such as flaring and intrusion. If the habit is already causing flaring, a Bluegrass appliance may be suggested. Ideally, addressing the habit before the permanent teeth erupt would be optimal, but it may not always be feasible.

HOW CAN I ENCOURAGE MY CHILD TO STOP THUMB-SUCKING?

To help children stop a thumb-sucking habit, it's important to consider their specific situation. If they are weaning themselves off the habit and the thumb falls out at night, then they will likely stop on their own. However, if the habit continues throughout the night and if one attempts pull the child's thumb out of their mouth, it causes their head to move with it, a habit appliance, such as a bluegrass appliance, may be recommended. This specific appliance is not intended to be removable. It is held in place with cemented orthodontic bands on the molars and an orthodontic wire runs behind the child's front teeth and supports a plastic bead which can be twirled with the tongue.

The intent is to replace the thumb-sucking habit with a distractor. It's important to explain the reasoning behind the appliance to the child and involve the child in the process. If a child is also interested in discontinuing the thumb sucking habit, but requires assistance, the therapy will be more effective. After six months of using the appliance, children often get bored with it and are ready to stop the habit. This personalized approach can be effective in helping children stop thumb-sucking without feeling embarrassed or ashamed.

HOW CAN I PREVENT MY CHILD FROM GRINDING THEIR TEETH AT NIGHT?

To help prevent a child from grinding their teeth at night first requires investigation into what might be the reason for the grinding. At times children will grind their teeth at night in response to stress, which may be physical, such as the onset of an illness or emotional stress. In these cases, grinding may be transient and resolve on its own. However, when a parent expresses concern about their child grinding their teeth, I will ask questions related to time of day, frequency, duration, quality of sleep, association with snoring and family history. Family history is relevant, because teeth grinding can be a symptom of airway concerns that may have anatomical origins (such as a tendency toward large tonsils or adenoids, or lowered smooth smooth muscle tone.) If there is suspicion that tooth grinding may be related to an anatomical concern, further investigation is needed and a collaborative approach to care is appropriate. An experienced ear, nose and throat specialist is a valuable team member when providing a collaborative approach to care.

WHAT ARE THE DANGERS OF SHARING UTENSILS AND DRINKS WITH MY CHILD?

The transmission of bacteria and viruses is a major concern. Sharing utensils and drinks can inoculate your child with a strain of cariogenic bacteria, which can cause cavities. Additionally, sharing utensils and drinks can also spread general illnesses. Cold sores, caused by a herpes virus, are transmitted through sharing utensils and drinks. Therefore, it's better to avoid sharing utensils and drinks with your child to prevent the transmission of bacteria and viruses.

HOW CAN I HELP MY CHILD AVOID JAW PROBLEMS?

To help avoid jaw problems which result in larger dental problems, it's important to maintain good oral hygiene habits, such as brushing twice a day, flossing regularly, and visiting the dentist for regular checkups and cleanings. Protecting the primary teeth aids in preventing future malocclusion, which can lead to jaw problems from an ill-fitting bite. Additionally, early evaluation by an orthodontist can identify and address any potential issues before they become more severe. While some dental problems may be unavoidable, following these preventive measures can help minimize the risk of extensive dental problems in the future.

HOW CAN I PREVENT DENTAL PROBLEMS IN MY CHILD WHILE THEY ARE SLEEPING?

To maintain good oral health, it's important to follow some basic habits. Firstly, make sure your child brushes their teeth before going to bed. Also, encourage them to drink water with their meals and whenever they feel thirsty during the night. This will help keep their mouth clean while they sleep. Additionally, it's best to avoid eating anything after brushing teeth, or if they do, choose something that's not cariogenic like an almond. If they need to wake up during the night to drink, make sure it's only water. Lastly, if you do have a child that is unable to sleep with their mouth closed, it is important to seek the advice of a pediatric dentist or a pediatrician. Mouth breathing can lead to an increased risk for dental decay, due to the dryness of the oral cavity that develops and prevents healthy saliva from keeping the children's teeth moist and remineralized. By following these simple practices, your child can maintain healthy teeth and avoid dental problems.

This is **ALPHA DENTISTRY vol. 3, PAEDIATRIC DENTISTRY FAQ**. Welcome to the Alphas.

Dr. BAK NGUYEN

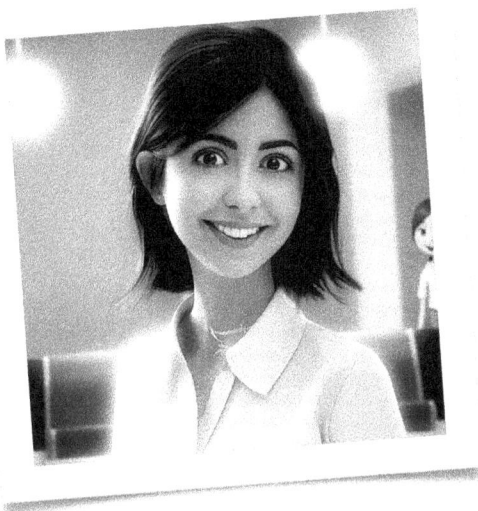

Dr. NIDHI TANEJA,

DDS, MSD

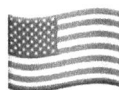

From the USA, **Dr. NIDHI TANEJA**, DDS, MSD, is a board-certified paediatric dentist. She is an expert in seeing children with special needs and those with dental fear and anxiety. She wants no child to ever be scared of going to the dentist. Her unique behaviour guidance and minimally invasive techniques, help children get through their dental visits with trust and confidence. After being in the conventional model of clinical dentistry which is heavily driven by procedures and surgical intervention, her goal is to help families and children experience dentistry without drills and fears. As a positive childhood advocate, she incorporates mindfulness-based principles in her practice for optimal oral and mental hygiene. She has been awarded 40 under 40 America's Best Dental Specialists, selected for Guiding Leaders program for Women Leadership and is actively involved in organized dentistry with the American Dental Association and the American Academy of Paediatric Dentistry.

I met Dr. Nidhi Taneja through the referral of our common friend, Dr. Richard Simpson. Dr. Taneja is the hope of the future of our profession. She is passionate, full of hope, and she has the energy to enlighten dentistry.

Yes, Nidhi is a paediatric dentist, a top 40 under 40, and full time clinician and an advocate of minimally invasive dentistry. She is great with kids and is passionate about preventive dentistry. Starting this book, I said that if we, the dental industry, should have to rebuild our public image, paediatric dentists should be the front people. Well, Nidhi surely embodies that hope.

For the last 25 years, I stood for a more humanized dentistry and will keep to do so. Well, collaborating with Dr. Taneja gave me the hope that the future is great and much brighter! Without further due, please join me to welcoming Dr. Nidhi Taneja.

This is **ALPHA DENTISTRY vol. 3, PAEDIATRIC DENTISTRY FAQ**. Welcome to the Alphas.

Dr. BAK NGUYEN

CHAPTER 5

"PAEDIATRIC DENTISTRY"

by Dr. NIDHI TANEJA

FROM USA

5.1 - DEFINITIONS

by Dr. NIDHI TANEJA FROM USA

WHAT IS THE BEST TYPE OF TOOTHBRUSH FOR MY CHILD?

When it comes to toothbrushes, different age groups may require different types of toothbrushes. For infants, a simple cleaning gauze or a clean piece of cloth wet with water to wipe the gums could be enough. For very young infants, silicone toothbrushes or finger toothbrushes can be used to clean the gums. As the child grows older, a small manual toothbrush can be gradually introduced with a head that is comfortable and does not hurt the gums or jaw bones while cleaning all surfaces of the teeth.

According to dental experts, the ideal age to introduce a toothbrush is around eight months when the first incisors upper and lower teeth appear. For children between the ages of zero and three, a small toothbrush can be used. Additionally, a three-sided toothbrush can be helpful for kids who struggle to spend more time brushing and for those with autism or special needs, as it can clean three surfaces of the teeth at once in a back-and-forth motion.

While electric toothbrushes have their advantages, it is recommended to start with a manual toothbrush to help the child get used to the proper brushing motion. Moreover, manual toothbrushes are easily portable and can be used anywhere. However, when using an electric toothbrush, it is crucial for parents to supervise the child and ensure that the bristles are kept on the teeth for a longer period of time instead of moving back and forth. Ultimately, both manual and electric toothbrushes can be equally efficient if used correctly.

WHAT IS THE ROLE OF FLUORIDE IN PREVENTING CAVITIES?

Fluoride has been shown in the literature to prevent cavities, with a mechanism of action that involves combining with the hydroxyapatite of the tooth structure and forming stronger fluorapatite molecules. Fluoride has also been found to be an antimicrobial against Streptococcus mutans, a primary bacteria that causes cavities. Studies have demonstrated that areas with fluoridated water have lower rates of cavities in children, making fluoride a helpful preventative measure for cavities.

WHAT IS THE DIFFERENCE BETWEEN A PAEDIATRIC DENTIST AND A GENERAL DENTIST?

A paediatric dentist is a specialist who treats children from birth to 21 years of age, as well as special needs adults. They receive additional training after obtaining their doctoral degree in dentistry, typically lasting two to three years, to specialize in children's dental care and advanced training in behavior management of children both pharmacologically and non-pharmacologically. Although general dentists may also treat children, paediatric dentists are dedicated specialists who exclusively focus on the dental needs of children.

WHAT ARE THE MOST COMMON ORTHODONTIC PROBLEMS IN CHILDREN?

There are several factors contributing to the increase in orthodontic referrals for children around six or seven years old. One of the main causes is oral habits like pacifier use and thumb-sucking, which can lead to a constricted upper jaw. Additionally, changes in the diet towards more processed and less fibrous foods that require less chewing can limit jaw growth, leading to tooth discrepancies and crowding. However, it's important to note that the size of the jaw is not just affected by growth hormones, but also by the utilization of the jaw muscles.

In ancient humans, for example, the jaw size was larger due to the utilization of these muscles through chewing fibrous foods. There is also evidence that the popularity of breastfeeding for less than two years old may be a contributing factor, as the natural growth of the jaw is stimulated through breastfeeding. Growth and development is multifactorial and a more thorough examination of the issue is needed from a morphological standpoint.

Regarding the distinction between the role of general dentists, and orthodontists, pediatric dentists typically see children at a very young age, starting from infancy up to around seven or eight years old when they take a panoramic X-ray to assess the status of the jaw and adult teeth. At this point, an orthodontist can take over with interceptive orthodontics, but pediatric dentists also perform a lot of interception at an earlier age using appliances like Invisalign First or Myo Munchies to develop the jaw utilizing the early natural growth potential. General dentists can also refer children to orthodontists at an appropriate time, but it's essential to note that both general and pediatric dentists can equally provide early intervention to detect problems and refer patients to the appropriate specialist.

HOW CAN I TELL IF MY CHILD NEEDS ORTHODONTIC TREATMENT?

I believe that the most effective way to monitor and evaluate the orthodontic needs of a child is through regular visits to the dentist. Paediatric dentists are specially trained to monitor the growth and development of the jaw and teeth, and they can assess how the teeth are coming in relation to the jaw growth. By visiting the dentist every six months, the dental age of the child can be monitored, and any potential orthodontic needs can be predicted and addressed early on. Therefore, whether you choose to see a paediatric dentist or a general dentist, regular dental visits are crucial for ensuring the optimal oral health and development of your child.

WHAT ARE THE BENEFITS OF DENTAL SEALANTS FOR CHILDREN?

Dental sealants are a protective coating that is applied to the grooves, pits, and fissures on the surface of adult and baby teeth to prevent food from getting trapped and causing cavities. This coating creates a smooth surface on the tooth, which makes it easier to clean and less likely to develop cavities. However, it is important to note that dental sealants do not guarantee that the tooth will never develop a cavity. To ensure that the sealant is effective, it must be applied to a cavity-free and clean tooth in a dry environment, using the appropriate techniques and materials to obtain a proper marginal seal.

Additionally, dental sealants can crack or break if the child bites down on hard objects like pencils or ice, and regular check-ups with the dentist every six months are necessary to ensure the sealant's integrity. If the dentist notices any breaks in the sealant, it may need to be replaced.

5.2 - PREVENTION

by Dr. NIDHI TANEJA FROM USA 🇺🇸

HOW CAN I PREPARE MY CHILD FOR THEIR FIRST DENTAL VISIT?

It is crucial to prepare children for their first dental visit as they may be experiencing a new and unfamiliar environment. They may even associate it with a medical visit, which can create fear and anxiety. It is recommended that parents take their child to the dentist by the age of one and prepare them by explaining the procedures beforehand. For instance, on their first visit, the dentist will examine their teeth, and parents can demonstrate this through video modelling, reading books, or showing cartoons. It is also advisable to schedule the visit in the morning when the child is alert and not tired. By taking these steps, parents can help make the first dental visit a positive experience for their child.

HOW CAN I HELP MY CHILD OVERCOME THEIR FEAR OF THE DENTIST?

There are several factors that can contribute to a child's dental anxiety and fear. One of them is biological, which means that the child may have inherent medical or sensory processing disorders that make them more fearful during a dental appointment. The other factor is environmental, which can include the child's exposure to dental fear through parents, siblings, or friends who may have talked about the dentist in a negative way or had a bad experience themselves.

It's crucial to take necessary precautions to ensure that the child's dental visits are as positive as possible, so that they do not develop fear or anxiety as they grow older. This can involve creating a welcoming and comfortable environment, using age-appropriate language to explain procedures, and encouraging the child's participation in their own dental care. By taking these steps, we can help children feel more confident and motivated to take care of their teeth.

HOW CAN I PREPARE MY CHILD FOR A DENTAL PROCEDURE?

While it's true that sugar is a necessary source of energy for the body, it's important to recognize that excessive sugar consumption can lead to negative health consequences, including dental issues such as cavities. From a dental perspective, the amount, frequency, and type of sugar consumed all play a role in oral health. It's crucial to avoid sugary snacks that can stick to teeth for prolonged periods of time, as this can increase the risk of tooth decay. It's also important for adults to help children clean their teeth after consuming sugary foods. While sugar isn't inherently bad, it's important to maintain a balanced diet and limit sugar consumption to ensure overall health and well-being.

IS IT OKAY FOR CHILDREN TO CONSUME SUGARY FOODS AND DRINKS?

One important point to keep in mind is that occasional indulgence in sweets is not harmful for a child's oral health as long as their teeth are properly cleaned afterwards. It's essential to maintain good oral hygiene habits like regular brushing and flossing, as well as rinsing the mouth with water after eating sugary snacks. This can help remove any remaining particles of food from the teeth and prevent them from causing decay.

Remember, sugary particles can get stuck in between teeth as well, so flossing is just as important as brushing. By incorporating these simple habits into their routine, children can enjoy sweets in moderation without compromising their dental health.

CAN MY CHILD STILL ENJOY SWEET TREATS WHILE MAINTAINING GOOD ORAL HYGIENE?

Yes, children can still enjoy sweet treats while maintaining good oral hygiene. The key is moderation and proper oral care. It's important to limit the frequency and amount of sugary snacks and beverages, and encourage children to brush and floss regularly. Additionally, parents can offer healthier snack options such as fruits and vegetables, and choose sugar-free gum or candies that are less likely to stick to the teeth. With proper oral care and moderation, children can enjoy sweet treats while keeping their teeth healthy.

HOW CAN I ENSURE MY CHILD IS RECEIVING ADEQUATE NUTRITION FOR HEALTHY TEETH?

When it comes to dental health, it's important to limit a child's exposure to sugar and fruit juices, as well as control the frequency of snacking. Nutritious foods like natural fruits and vegetables, nuts, milk, and unrefined sugars should be encouraged instead. As for the claim that milk and cheese are good for teeth, some milk products contain calcium which is important for the formation of teeth, but lactose-intolerant children may need to get their calcium from other sources. A paediatrician can help ensure that children are getting the necessary nutrients for healthy teeth.

HOW CAN I PREVENT ORTHODONTIC PROBLEMS IN MY CHILD?

It is crucial for us to monitor a child's growth as some orthodontic problems are not preventable due to genetics. For example, if a child inherits smaller teeth genes from the mother and larger jaw genes from the father, their smile may appear straight. However, if it is the opposite and the child has a smaller jaw from the mother and larger teeth genes from the father, there may be a discrepancy. While genetics play a significant role in orthodontic problems, we can still control some factors such as early use of pacifiers, thumb-sucking, and other non-nutritive oral habits. We need to ensure that children break these habits at the right age.

5.3 - TIME

by Dr. NIDHI TANEJA FROM USA

WHAT IS THE BEST AGE FOR A CHILD TO START SEEING A DENTIST?

The American Academy of Paediatric Dentistry recommends that a child should have their first dental visit by the age of one, or when their first tooth erupts, whichever comes first. The first tooth usually appears around six months of age, but this can vary from child to child. Therefore, it is important for parents to schedule their child's first dental appointment by age one, regardless of whether or not their child has a tooth yet.

HOW OFTEN SHOULD MY CHILD SEE A DENTIST?

Regular visits to the dentist every six months are recommended for two important reasons. Firstly, it allows the dentist to catch any potential disease process early on and educate parents on how to prevent such conditions from occurring. Secondly, it helps young children become accustomed to going to the dentist regularly, reducing their fear and anxiety towards future dental visits. By establishing a routine of regular dental check-ups from an early age, children are more likely to maintain good oral health throughout their lives.

WHAT IS THE BEST AGE FOR A CHILD TO GET ORTHODONTIC TREATMENT?

Every child is unique, and if a paediatric dentist notices an issue early on, there are interception methods that can be applied before the child reaches seven years of age, such as breaking off bad habits. However, in most cases, significant changes can be detected around the age of seven, when the first permanent molars and incisors have fully erupted, allowing for the prediction of jaw growth. Since children are still in their growth phase, this period can be utilized to prevent severe crowding or other issues. Therefore, we typically recommend seeing an orthodontist around the age of seven.

One of the most commonly used devices for orthodontic treatment is a maxillary expander. This device is used when the child is still growing and their maxillary sutures have not yet fused, which usually occurs before puberty. By applying pressure, the expander can induce the expansion of the jaw, creating more space for the teeth and helping them come into better alignment. This technique is especially effective in cases where teeth are impacted or overcrowded. Once the child's maxillary sutures have fused, inducing growth becomes much more challenging. However, some studies have shown that inducing growth is possible in adults as well, though it is generally more difficult than in children.

WHAT ARE THE SIGNS OF TEETH ERUPTION IN A CHILD?
When a child's teeth are erupting, there are several signs that parents can look out for. One common indicator is a bulge where the new tooth is pushing through the gums. Another sign is the presence of an eruption hematoma, which appears as a bluish tinge caused by the blood vessels inside the gums rupturing due to the pressure of the emerging tooth. In some cases, there may be swelling or discomfort in the area for the first few days.

Children may also drool excessively or put objects in their mouth to relieve the pressure sensation. As for fever, it is not typically associated with tooth eruption, despite what some people may believe. If a child does experience a fever during this time, it is important to consult with a paediatrician to determine the underlying cause. While irritation from erupting teeth may contribute to fever, it is not a direct symptom of tooth eruption.

5.4 - MAINTENANCE
by Dr. NIDHI TANEJA FROM USA

WHAT IS THE RIGHT WAY TO CLEAN MY CHILD'S TEETH?
Proper oral hygiene involves cleaning all surfaces of the teeth, which are divided into five sections: the chewing

surface, the inside surface (toward the tongue), the outside surface (toward the lips/cheeks), and the two sides where the teeth touch each other. Brushing should be done in circular motions at the area where the teeth and gums meet, and all five surfaces of the teeth should be cleaned. Flossing is also essential to reach the spaces in between the teeth. Both brushing and flossing are necessary for good oral hygiene. It is recommended to brush your teeth for two minutes, twice a day. For younger children with fewer teeth, the time can be shorter, around 40 seconds. It is important to use a toothbrush appropriate for a child's age and size and to ensure that all surfaces of the teeth are properly cleaned.

HOW CAN I ENCOURAGE MY CHILD TO BRUSH THEIR TEETH REGULARLY?

One of the most important things to establish good oral hygiene is to introduce the habit early on and not give up if the child resists. It's important to make toothbrushing a part of their natural routine and hygiene habits. Good modelling at home is also important, and children should see their parents brushing. Using timers, alarms, or reward charts can also encourage children to brush regularly. Making toothbrushing a fun experience for children can be helpful, such as asking them questions or giving them choices while brushing. If children are resistant, it can be helpful to treat toothbrushing like changing a diaper - a necessary task that must be done consistently. It's important to be gentle but firm and not give up, especially during the early years when a child's comprehension is still developing.

HOW CAN I PREVENT TOOTH DECAY IN MY CHILD'S BABY TEETH?

Maintaining good oral health involves three important practices. The first is having a healthy diet, which includes limiting sugary foods and drinks. The second is building a regular toothbrushing habit, brushing twice a day in the morning and at night. And the third is regularly visiting the dentist every six months. By doing so, any potential problems can be detected early on, and both parents and children can be educated on proper oral hygiene practices. Remember, a good diet, regular toothbrushing, and dental check-ups every six months are crucial for maintaining good oral health.

HOW CAN I PREVENT MY CHILD FROM DEVELOPING DENTAL ANXIETY?

It is crucial for children to be exposed to dental visits in a non-threatening way as early as possible before any disease processes begin. Paediatric dentists aim to make dental visits fun and prevention-focused. By exposing children to the dentist's office before any pain or cavities develop, the first visit can be easy and friendly, with just a teeth cleaning and education on the importance of toothbrushing and nutrition. However, if the child already has a cavity, the procedure can be more invasive and potentially traumatic, depending on the severity of the disease. Therefore, it is important to see the dentist early on to prevent the need for more extensive procedures in the first place or find an appropriate mode of sedation to assist in restoring to dental health.

HOW CAN I HELP MY CHILD AVOID DENTAL INJURIES?

Different age groups have different dental care recommendations. For very young children, it is important to take care of their environment and ensure that they are not exposed to any potential hazards that can harm their teeth. For teenagers, it is crucial to wear mouth guards when playing sports, especially because they have permanent teeth that need protection. We also advise children not to use their teeth to open soda cans or chip packets as this can cause damage to their teeth. It is essential to supervise young children and prevent them from being in an environment that can cause injury, such as falling or hitting concrete accidentally.

HOW CAN I HELP MY CHILD AVOID GUM DISEASE?

Gums are an essential part of our oral cavity and need to be cared for along with our teeth. When we use circular motions while brushing our teeth, the gums also receive a massage, and the cell turnover helps keep them clean. Warm salt water rinses can also be used occasionally to ensure our gums and teeth are well rinsed. While flossing is typically used when teeth are in contact, it's recommended to start flossing around age two, regardless of whether teeth are touching or not. This habit can be encouraged by parents modelling flossing and reminding each other to floss. Dentists will inform parents when their child's baby teeth start touching and it's time to floss regularly. It's also interesting to note that assigning children the task of reminding their parents to floss can be an effective strategy.

HOW CAN I HELP MY CHILD MAINTAIN GOOD ORAL HYGIENE WHILE WEARING BRACES?

When a child has braces or any oral appliances, there is an increased risk of food debris getting stuck around them, which can lead to cavities. Therefore, it's important to take extra time to clean around the braces and limit the consumption of sugary drinks and sticky foods that can easily get stuck. It is also recommended to use a Waterpik to clean areas where the toothbrush cannot reach, especially in cases where the gums are very tight around the braces. By following these practices, children can maintain good oral hygiene and prevent any complications during their orthodontic treatment.

HOW CAN I HELP MY CHILD AVOID TOOTH SENSITIVITY?

It is important to help young children avoid tooth sensitivity, as their teeth are still developing their hard enamel and dentin, which makes them more sensitive to extremes of temperature. Using Sensodyne toothpaste can be helpful if they experience sensitivity. It is also recommended to avoid acidic foods and drinks, such as soda and carbonated drinks, which can create an acidic environment that can dissolve tooth structure and make it more porous.

5.5 - DENTAL WORK

by Dr. NIDHI TANEJA FROM USA 🇺🇸

WHAT ARE THE MOST COMMON DENTAL PROBLEMS IN CHILDREN?

Dental caries is one of the most common and chronic childhood diseases in America. It is caused by a complex interplay between the microbiome, the tooth structure, and diet. While it may be difficult to create a chart that fully explains the etiology of dental caries, it is important for parents to understand the factors that contribute to the development of this disease in order to prevent it.

WHAT CAN I DO IF MY CHILD HAS A DENTAL EMERGENCY?

It is important to establish a dental home for your child, which is a relationship with a dentist in your area. This way, in case of a dental emergency, you can call your dentist or go to a hospital with dental employees. In the case of a minor tooth injury, your dentist can triage it and recommend palliative treatment. If your dentist is unable to provide emergency treatment, it may be necessary to go to the hospital for dental care.

IS IT NECESSARY FOR MY CHILD TO HAVE DENTAL X-RAYS TAKEN?

X-rays are an essential tool for dentists to diagnose dental issues that are not visible to the naked eye. They are particularly helpful for detecting cavities in between teeth and checking for abnormalities in the development of adult teeth. It is important to take X-rays to catch these issues early and promote long-term oral health. X-rays are typically recommended when teeth start to touch, and in my practice, we recommend X-rays after the age of four. However, in the case of trauma or fractures, we may take limited X-rays even in younger children. It is important to note that X-rays are safe and pose minimal risk when proper precautions are taken.

WHAT IS THE BEST WAY TO TREAT A CHILD'S CAVITIES?

At this stage, there are numerous options available to restore dental caries to the satisfaction of parents. In the past, we used amalgams, which are silver fillings. However, more recently, we use white fillings made of composites and glass ionomer fillings. Both of these materials are white and successful in children. Glass ionomer fillings have the advantage of being less technique-sensitive and release fluoride, which has a preventive aspect. Depending on the size of the cavity, we may also use stainless steel crowns to prevent the filling from fracturing in case of large cavities.

WHAT IS DENTAL SEALANT, AND IS IT NECESSARY FOR MY CHILD?

As previously discussed, dental sealants are a preventative procedure that can be very beneficial for children with deep grooves in their teeth. These grooves can make it difficult to clean the teeth, and sealants can make them self-cleansing and reduce the risk of cavities. There are no known harmful effects of getting sealants, as long as the child is able to tolerate the procedure and they are done with proper technique and under isolation.

However, it can be expensive if insurance does not cover it. Sealants are typically not necessary for baby teeth and may not be needed after a certain age if the grooves are not deep or if the tooth has been cavity-free. The cost of sealants in the United States ranges from $40 to $70, which is significantly less expensive than getting a cavity filled. Many insurances cover this as a preventive benefit.

WHAT ARE THE BENEFITS OF ORTHODONTIC TREATMENT FOR CHILDREN?

Orthodontic treatment can help align teeth to improve both their aesthetic appearance and their functionality. Proper alignment can make teeth easier to clean, reducing the risk of food particles getting stuck and the subsequent risk of cavities. Additionally, good alignment can improve occlusion, reducing the risk of trauma to the teeth. Treatment can also boost a child's morale by improving their smile and overall oral health. By investing in orthodontic treatment, parents can help ensure the long-term preservation of their child's teeth.

IS IT OKAY FOR MY CHILD TO PLAY SPORTS WITH BRACES?
Yes, children can play sports while wearing braces, but it is important to use a mouth guard to protect their teeth. Mouth guards are especially crucial for contact sports that involve a high risk of abrasion or injury to the mouth. So it is important to make sure that the child wears a mouth guard during contact sports.

WHAT ARE THE RISKS OF NOT TREATING MY CHILD'S CAVITIES?
Our teeth are a crucial part of our body and their health is connected to our overall systemic health. If we neglect a dental cavity, it's like keeping an infection in your mouth that can affect your entire body. If we don't treat the cavity in its early stages and maintain good oral hygiene, it will continue to grow and increase the risk of harmful bacteria in the mouth. This can not only make other teeth more susceptible to cavities, but it can also lead to systemic infections such as abscesses. Ultimately, we may have to extract the tooth due to pain and infection if the cavity is left untreated.

HOW CAN I PREVENT BABY BOTTLE TOOTH DECAY IN MY CHILD?
Cavities in baby teeth, also known as early childhood caries, are more common in young children who are breastfed throughout the night or consume milk from a bottle before sleeping. This is because the frequent exposure of the teeth to milk, which breaks down into sugar, can lead to the growth of bacteria that cause

tooth decay. To prevent this, it is important to clean the child's teeth after they have had their milk and gradually wean them off the habit. Additionally, an adult can clean the child's teeth while they are sleeping to remove any milk residue. This helps to ensure that the child's teeth are protected from the harmful effects of milk sugar and bacteria.

HOW CAN I FIND A PAEDIATRIC DENTIST FOR MY CHILD?

The internet can be a helpful tool to find paediatric dentists in your area. In the United States, the American Academy of Paediatric Dentistry provides a centralized platform for certified dentists. However, with a simple online search, you can easily find a dentist in your region. Regarding finding a good dentist, it's essential to choose a paediatric dentist who can establish a positive connection with you and your child. You should feel comfortable asking questions, and the dentist should provide satisfactory answers. Additionally, the dentist should create a non-threatening environment to make your child feel safe and happy. If you feel that your child's needs are not being met, it's okay to discuss your concerns with the dentist and explore other options until you find the right fit.

HOW CAN I HELP MY CHILD MAINTAIN GOOD ORAL HYGIENE WHILE WEARING APPLIANCES?

It's important to note that any oral appliance, including braces, can harbour bacteria. To prevent this, it's crucial for children to rinse their mouth after every meal and keep a toothbrush with them, even when they're at school, to brush away any food particles that may get stuck around their braces or appliances. As adults, we can supervise and help them regularly to ensure their appliances are kept clean.

5.6 - FEAR/PAIN

by Dr. NIDHI TANEJA FROM USA 🇺🇸

IS SEDATION DENTISTRY NECESSARY FOR CHILDREN?

Sedation for dental appointments is determined on a case-by-case basis. Typically, sedation is not necessary for non-restorative appointments. However, if a child has had a bad experience in the past, is uncooperative, or has severe dental needs, mild or moderate sedation may be necessary. General anesthesia is sometimes recommended if it is safe for the child. The goal is to eliminate any disease process in a safe and non-traumatic way, and often this means sedation is required. The risk and appropriate age for sedation should be discussed with a dental anesthesiologist or anesthesiologist. Laughing gas is a safe and simple option for mild sedation and can be used as early as two years old. However, sedation is only used when necessary to increase the child's pain tolerance and make the appointment more comfortable.

HOW CAN I HELP MY CHILD COPE WITH TOOTH LOSS?

We love it when children around the age of six come in and have a loose tooth. We often have them tell us about the Tooth Fairy, who is said to leave a prize for children who have clean teeth. This helps them to understand that losing teeth is a normal part of growing up, and they may even see their friends experiencing the same thing. We think it's important to make these experiences fun and enjoyable, so we always try to incorporate playful elements like the Tooth Fairy story.

HOW CAN I RELIEVE MY CHILD'S TOOTH ERUPTION PAIN?

Tooth eruption can be uncomfortable for children due to the pressure of the new tooth. Instead of using over-the-counter medication or gel, a small drop of vegetable oil or vitamin E oil can be massaged on the gums for relief. Cold towels, teething toys, or spoons can also be used temporarily to alleviate the pain. If a child is still uncomfortable, over-the-counter pain medicine for kids can be given.

WHAT ARE THE RISKS OF USING TEETHING GELS AND CREAMS?

I generally advise against using teething gels and creams as they can be considered unnecessary medication for the child with no significant benefits. Additionally, it is difficult to control the dosage of such products, so I do not recommend them.

HOW CAN I HELP MY CHILD RECOVER AFTER A DENTAL PROCEDURE?

Sometimes a child has a positive experience at the dentist, which makes them excited to return. Good communication and positive feedback can help with this. However, there are times when a child has a negative experience, especially in emergencies or when they are uncooperative. After the procedure, it's important to explain to the child why it was necessary and how it will help them. We can also help them cope with anxiety by listening to their concerns and communicating future appointments. Building good habits at home is also important. It's our hope that after any emergency procedure, the child will return for regular, non-invasive visits, which can help eliminate any bad experiences from the past.

WHAT IS THE COST OF PAEDIATRIC DENTAL CARE?

Paediatric dental care is not significantly cheaper than adult care, despite the fact that we focus mainly on prevention and baby teeth, which will impact the permanent teeth. While preventive care is usually covered by dental insurance in America, it can still be a financial burden for some parents.

ARE THOSE COVERED BY THE GOVERNMENT?

The coverage for paediatric dentistry in the United States varies depending on the insurance plan and government programs available. While some government programs may provide coverage for preventive and some procedural care for children up to the age of 21, coverage is also influenced by the socioeconomic status of the parents. However, there are still challenges in accessing dental care, particularly in areas with lower socioeconomic status, where there may be a shortage of dentists. Therefore, despite the availability of coverage, accessing dental care remains a challenge for some families.

ARE INSURANCE COVERING CHILD DENTAL CARE?

Yes, the majority of dental insurance plans provide coverage for preventive procedures for children.

5.8 - HABITS

by Dr. NIDHI TANEJA FROM USA 🇺🇸

IS THUMB-SUCKING HARMFUL TO MY CHILD'S TEETH?

Non-nutritive sucking, such as thumb sucking, can be harmful to a child's dental health. While it may provide comfort initially, once teeth begin to erupt, the pressure of the thumb can narrow the upper jaw and change the shape of the palate, which can lead to arch length discrepancy and an increased risk of crowding. This can ultimately result in the need for braces in the future. It is important to discourage thumb-sucking as early as possible to prevent these dental problems.

HOW CAN I ENCOURAGE MY CHILD TO STOP THUMB-SUCKING?

There are different strategies that I recommend to parents to help their child stop thumb-sucking. First and foremost, it is important to have an open and honest conversation with the child about breaking the habit. Some methods that can be used to facilitate this include having the child wear an oversized long sleeve shirt at night and tying the ends of the sleeves together so that the hand is not exposed. Another option is to use a thumb guard or Band-Aid as a reminder. Additionally, parents can create a habit-breaking chart or game for their child, where they can earn stars or rewards for every day that they don't suck their thumb. These positive reinforcements can motivate the child and make breaking the habit more fun and engaging.

HOW CAN I PREVENT MY CHILD FROM GRINDING THEIR TEETH AT NIGHT?

I understand your concern about your child's teeth grinding. While there is currently no concrete way to break the habit in young children, we can look into social factors such as stress and anxiety as potential triggers. It's important to monitor your child's grinding and check for any detrimental signs on the teeth. If there are signs of damage, we can provide a mouth guard to protect the teeth while the habit is being addressed. It's also helpful to talk to your child and try to identify any potential sources of stress or anxiety. If the habit persists, we can continue to monitor it and work with you to find solutions.

WHAT ARE THE DANGERS OF SHARING UTENSILS AND DRINKS WITH MY CHILD?

It is important to note that disease transfer can occur vertically or horizontally. In the case of bad oral health and microbiome in parents, it is possible for the child to inherit these issues. Similarly, siblings can also share bacteria through tonsils and utensils, which can lead to the spread of active cavities or other oral health problems. It's important to be aware of these potential sources of disease transfer and take steps to prevent them, such as practicing good oral hygiene and avoiding sharing utensils with those who have active dental issues.

HOW CAN I HELP MY CHILD AVOID JAW PROBLEMS?

I understand your concern about jaw problems and occlusion. Early intervention is key to preventing any potential issues. When a dentist notices a jaw discrepancy at a young age, there are more opportunities to prevent it by intervening early and utilizing the child's growth. Harmful oral habits should be eliminated at an earlier age to prevent any malocclusion problems from worsening. Genetic factors may be beyond our control, but we can still take steps to prevent any potential issues. Therefore, it is recommended to get the child checked by a dentist early on to identify and potentially address any jaw problems.

HOW CAN I PREVENT DENTAL PROBLEMS IN MY CHILD WHILE THEY ARE SLEEPING?

I can suggest two common habits that can harm a child's oral health. The first is thumb-sucking, which many children tend to do, especially while sleeping. The second is early childhood decay, which can occur when a child drinks from a bottle before bedtime. As we discussed earlier, it is important to ensure that the child does not consume any food or drinks before going to bed and that the last thing that touches their teeth is water. Additionally, it is crucial to establish a good routine of brushing their teeth before bedtime.

This is **ALPHA DENTISTRY vol. 3, PAEDIATRIC DENTISTRY FAQ**. Welcome to the Alphas.

Dr. BAK NGUYEN

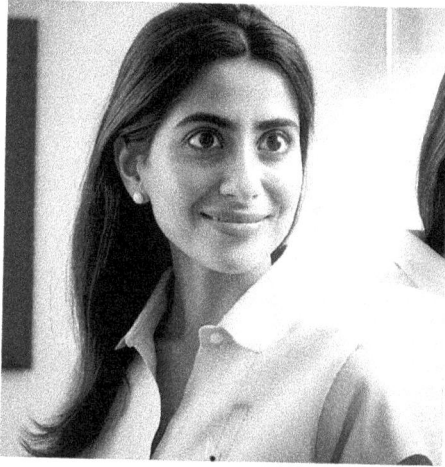

Dr. AURORA ALVA,
DMD

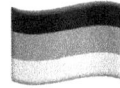

From GERMANY , **Dr. AURORA ALVA**, DMD, is an American board-certified paediatric dentist, a member of the American College of Paediatric Dentists, and a diplomate of the American Board of Paediatric Dentists. She started her career by obtaining a Biology degree from Wellesley College in Wellesley, Massachusetts, where she graduated Cum Laude. During her time at Wellesley, she also had the opportunity to successfully complete courses at the Massachusetts Institute of Technology (MIT) and immersed herself in summer research projects at Harvard Medical School. She obtained various college stipends for her achievements, such as from the Howard Hughes Medical Institute, and upon graduation, was one of the two recipients of the Wellesley College Graduate Fellowship Award. She obtained her dental degree and Pediatric Dentistry certificate from Tufts School of Dental Medicine in Boston, Massachusetts in 2007 and 2009, respectively. Dr. Alva's pediatric dental professional career has been diverse. She has worked in private practice in Massachusetts, Texas, and Georgia, participated in humanitarian dental missions in Honduras and Ecuador, worked as a pediatric dental contractor for the American Army in Germany, and worked in private practices in Munich, Germany. Dr. Aurora Alva holds professional licenses from the states of Georgia, Texas, Hawaii, California, and the region of Bavaria in Germany. She is an active member of the American Dental Association, the American Academy of Paediatric Dentists, and the American Board of Paediatric Dentists.

Dr. Aurora Alva and I go back to the beginning of this endeavor, the dream to democratize dental medicine, back in 2021. I was introduced to Aurora by a common friend and Alpha, Dr. Paul Dominique. Well, it did not take long to ignite Aurora's passion to join the Alphas.

I was happy to find an international expert who has experience in 2 countries, USA and Germany, But that was an understatement. Within weeks, we grew closer to becoming friends and partners. Since then, Dr. Alva is amongst the most active Alphas, helping me in recruiting more international KOLs to our series of books and endeavours.

Dr. Nour Ammar, Dr. Pierluigi Peligalli, and Dr. Ailin Cabrera-Matta are Alphas thanks to Dr. Alva intervention. In ALPHA 1, Dr. Judith Baumler has also been introduced by Dr. Alva. In simple words, Dr. Alva contributed, not only as a co-author, but also to spreading the influence of the ALPHAS in Europe and South America.

Always calm and smiling, Aurora, you are the kind friend who helps me believe when I am tired. You are the enthusiasm of the team when faced with waiting and doubts. Thank you for your trust and friendship. I am in your debt. Thank you for being a wonderful friend, a passionate doctor, and an engaged Alpha. Without further due, please join me in welcoming back, Alpha Dentist, Dr. Aurora Alva.

This is **ALPHA DENTISTRY vol. 3, PAEDIATRIC DENTISTRY FAQ**. Welcome to the Alphas.

CHAPTER 6

"PAEDIATRIC DENTISTRY"

by Dr. AURORA ALVA

FROM GERMANY

6.1 - DEFINITIONS

by Dr. AURORA ALVA FROM GERMANY

WHAT IS THE BEST TYPE OF TOOTHBRUSH FOR MY CHILD?

When it comes to selecting the best toothbrush for children, it is important to consider their preferences and needs. The key factor to keep in mind is choosing a toothbrush that they will actually use. It is recommended to select a toothbrush that is designed for their age, with soft bristles and a small head that can effectively clean all tooth surfaces, including the hard-to-reach areas in the back of the mouth. Electric toothbrushes can also be a great option for children because they have been proven to more efficiently remove plaque compared to manual toothbrushes. Electric toothbrushes can make brushing more fun and engaging for children, increasing their motivation to brush regularly. Ultimately, the best toothbrush for a child is one that they are comfortable using and that can effectively clean their teeth.

WHAT IS THE ROLE OF FLUORIDE IN PREVENTING CAVITIES?

Fluoride is a mineral that can help strengthen tooth enamel and even reverse early signs of tooth decay when it is applied directly on the surface of the teeth. This can be achieved by using fluoride toothpaste every day and by receiving fluoride treatments from the dentist. It is essential to use the right amount of fluoride toothpaste to avoid a condition called fluorosis, which can happen when someone consumes too much fluoride. For children under three years old, a small smear of toothpaste is enough, while older children should use a pea-sized amount to make sure they get the benefits of fluoride without any risks.

WHAT IS THE DIFFERENCE BETWEEN A PAEDIATRIC DENTIST AND A GENERAL DENTIST?

Pediatric dentists are dental specialists who have received specialized training in treating children of all ages. They are experts in managing the unique dental needs and behaviors of children, which can be very different from those of adults. Pediatric dentists are equipped with a wide range of behavior management techniques, which can help make a child's visit to the dentist a positive experience. These techniques can include various forms of sedation, such as nitrous oxide (laughing gas), oral sedatives, or general anesthesia, to help children relax and feel comfortable during dental procedures.

Additionally, pediatric dentists may use special equipment and tools designed specifically for children, as well as techniques for communicating with children effectively. While general dentists are also capable of treating children, pediatric dentists have received additional training and education that make them better equipped to handle complex cases involving both treatment and behavior management. As a result, some general dentists may refer very young children or those who require extensive treatment to pediatric dentists to ensure they receive the best possible care.

WHAT ARE THE MOST COMMON ORTHODONTIC PROBLEMS IN CHILDREN?

Pediatric dentists commonly encounter orthodontic problems in children, such as crowded teeth, finger habits, and misaligned teeth. If the problem is severe or complex, patients can be referred to an orthodontist. Pediatric dentists can provide basic orthodontic treatments like habit-breaker appliances and space maintenance procedures to intervene early and prevent more serious orthodontic issues.

HOW CAN I TELL IF MY CHILD NEEDS ORTHODONTIC TREATMENT?

Orthodontic problems in children, such as crowded teeth, open bites, and delayed tooth eruption, can have visible signs. However, some issues like asymmetric tooth eruption or baby teeth not falling out at the right time may not be noticeable right away. Pediatric dentists check for these problems during recall appointments and can identify them for early intervention.

WHAT ARE THE BENEFITS OF DENTAL SEALANTS FOR CHILDREN?

Sealants are a protective coating that can be applied to the chewing surfaces of back teeth. They work by filling in the grooves and pits on the tooth surface, creating a smooth surface that is easier to clean. This reduces the risk of cavities by preventing food particles and bacteria from getting trapped in these hard-to-reach areas. Sealants are suitable for both baby and permanent teeth, and they are a simple and painless procedure that can be done by a dentist. It is important to understand that while sealants can provide significant protection against cavities, they do not guarantee complete prevention. The level of protection varies depending on individual risk factors such as diet and oral hygiene habits. For this reason, it is essential to maintain good oral hygiene practices and visit the dentist regularly for checkups and cleanings.

6.2 - PREVENTION

by Dr. AURORA ALVA FROM GERMANY ▄

HOW CAN I PREPARE MY CHILD FOR THEIR FIRST DENTAL VISIT?

When children have an idea of what will happen during a dental visit, they are typically more willing to cooperate. For a basic cleaning and exam, parents can prepare their child by explaining that they will need to open their mouth wide and remain still. It is also helpful to discuss the various tools that the dentist will use, such as a mirror and a special toothbrush to clean all of their teeth. To promote good behavior, positive reinforcement and rewards can be effective strategies. Parents are essential in making their child feel at ease during dental visits. By collaborating with the dental team, we can ensure that your child has a successful and pleasant experience.

HOW CAN I HELP MY CHILD OVERCOME THEIR FEAR OF THE DENTIST?

Building trust is key to helping a child overcome their fear of the dentist. This effort involves parents, staff, and dentists working together. Often fear is based on not knowing what may happen so it is best to familiarize the child with dental procedures step by step. For their first appointment, I would suggest starting with a cleaning and evaluation so they can get used to the "dentist tools," the sounds, and meeting the dentist and staff. If the child has a cavity that needs to be filled, and there is no pain, I suggest starting with the smallest cavity that will not require a shot. For future filling appointments, if a shot may be needed, offering simple explanations like "the dentist will use a sleepy juice to make your teeth go to sleep" can be helpful.

To ensure a positive dental experience for your child, it is important to be a supportive ally during appointments and remain calm and confident. Children can easily pick up on a parent's mistrust or fear, so it is best to avoid comments such as "I am here to protect you" or "I will not let them do anything bad to you." Instead, use words that encourage trust, such as "the dentist and their team are here to help you have healthy teeth so you can eat without any pain." By building trust over time, your child can learn to see the dentist as a friend who helps keep their teeth healthy and pain-free.

HOW CAN I PREPARE MY CHILD FOR A DENTAL PROCEDURE?
Children have better cooperation when they know in advance what may happen. It will be a good idea to talk in advance about the dentist's tools that will be used such as the mirror or the special spinning toothbrush. Also, speak about how the dentist and the staff are there to help them have healthy teeth. On our side, we will explain all the tools we will be using and also approach the child in a kind and friendly manner to have a successful outcome.

IS IT OKAY FOR CHILDREN TO CONSUME SUGARY FOODS AND DRINKS?
The consumption of frequent sugary foods and drinks, especially outside of mealtimes, increases the risk of

developing cavities. I suggest limiting the intake of sugary foods and drinks, particularly at a young age.

CAN MY CHILD STILL ENJOY SWEET TREATS WHILE MAINTAINING GOOD ORAL HYGIENE?

It is possible for your child to enjoy sweet treats without negatively impacting their oral health, as long as those treats are healthier options like fruits. It is important to maintain good oral hygiene practices, particularly if the treat is consumed right before bedtime. This is because the risk of developing cavities is higher during the night, so make sure your child brushes their teeth before going to bed.

HOW CAN I ENSURE MY CHILD IS RECEIVING ADEQUATE NUTRITION FOR HEALTHY TEETH?

Baby teeth are more susceptible to cavities than permanent teeth because they have thinner enamel, which makes them more vulnerable to decay. To help prevent cavities, it is essential to limit your child's intake of sugary foods and drinks, especially in between meals. Choosing natural foods and water instead of sugary drinks can help promote good oral health.

HOW CAN I ENSURE MY CHILD IS GETTING ENOUGH FLUORIDE?

Nowadays, we get fluoride from various sources, including fluoride-fortified powdered milk for babies, foods prepared with fluoridated water, toothpaste with fluoride, and water in fluoridated communities. If the child lives in a non-fluoridated community parents should consult with their dentist regarding the need for a fluoride supplement.

HOW CAN I PREVENT ORTHODONTIC PROBLEMS IN MY CHILD?

Orthodontic problems can arise from various factors such as genetics or habits like thumb-sucking. If these habits are not stopped early, they may cause issues like open bite, crossbite, or crowding. While some orthodontic issues, such as spacing problems, may be inherited and cannot be prevented, it is important to address the preventable factors early on. Parents can ensure early detection of dental problems by taking their children for regular dental check-ups. This way, any orthodontic issues can be detected early and treated before they become more severe.

6.3 - TIME

by Dr. AURORA ALVA FROM GERMANY

WHAT IS THE BEST AGE FOR A CHILD TO START SEEING A DENTIST?

When a child's first tooth appears, usually around six months old, it is recommended to establish a dental home where the child can receive regular dental check-ups. These appointments are an opportunity for parents to ask questions and receive guidance on how to care for their child's teeth and gums. This includes information on topics such as teething, proper brushing techniques, nutrition, dental injuries, and avoiding harmful habits such as thumb-sucking. Even if the child does not have any teeth yet, these early appointments can provide valuable advice for parents to anticipate and prepare for their child's dental needs.

HOW OFTEN SHOULD MY CHILD SEE A DENTIST?

I recommend that parents bring their children for check-ups every six months so that we can monitor their oral health and make adjustments to their oral care routine as needed. If I notice inadequate oral hygiene or the presence of cavities, I would recommend that the child comes for check-ups every three months.

WHAT IS THE BEST AGE FOR A CHILD TO GET ORTHODONTIC TREATMENT?

Orthodontic referral is usually recommended around the age of 7 or 8 when the four front teeth and permanent molars on each side have come in. At this age, the orthodontist can evaluate the child's dental development and identify any potential problems with the bite or tooth alignment. However, in some cases, an earlier referral may be necessary based on the child's teeth development or the bite condition.

WHAT ARE THE SIGNS OF TEETH ERUPTION IN A CHILD?

The signs of teething can differ among children. While some may experience gum pain, swelling, or a change in gum color, others may drool excessively or have disrupted sleep.

6.4 - MAINTENANCE

by Dr. AURORA ALVA FROM GERMANY

WHAT IS THE RIGHT WAY TO CLEAN MY CHILD'S TEETH?

To make sure your child's teeth are well-cleaned, it's important to brush all sides of their teeth - the front, back, and sides. Don't forget to clean the tongue too, as it can harbor bacteria that cause bad breath and other oral health problems. Often, kids may skip brushing their tongue, so make sure to remind them to do so regularly.

HOW CAN I ENCOURAGE MY CHILD TO BRUSH THEIR TEETH REGULARLY?

There are several methods you can try to encourage your child to brush their teeth regularly. For example, you can make it a fun family activity by brushing together. You can also use a timer to turn brushing into a game, offer rewards for consistent brushing, and let them choose fun toothbrushes and toothpaste. Additionally, establishing a daily routine, teaching them about the importance of oral hygiene, and ensuring they attend regular dental check-ups are all great ways to motivate them.

However, there may be cases where children, especially young ones, may resist brushing their teeth for various reasons. In such situations, parents or guardians should work together as a team and make every effort to brush all of their child's teeth. During the child's first dental visit, the pediatric dentist can demonstrate how to accomplish this.

HOW CAN I PREVENT TOOTH DECAY IN MY CHILD'S BABY TEETH?

Brushing with fluoride toothpaste at least twice a day and avoiding sugary intake outside of mealtimes can decrease the chances of developing cavities. To achieve this, parents can encourage their children to have three satisfying meals a day, which eliminates the need for snacks outside of meal times. When thirsty, children should be offered water instead of sugary drinks or juices. Although vitamins are important for a child's health, some chewy vitamins may contain high levels of sugar, which can contribute to tooth decay. Regular dental visits can also help ensure early detection and appropriate treatment of any dental issues.

HOW CAN I PREVENT MY CHILD FROM DEVELOPING DENTAL ANXIETY?

It is important to find a dentist and dental office where your child feels comfortable. Look for a friendly and patient staff that can put your child at ease. Also, some children may be more anxious than others. If your child experiences anxiety during a routine cleaning, more complex treatments may be even more challenging. In such cases, options like laughing gas, oral sedation, or general anesthesia will be more helpful.

HOW CAN I HELP MY CHILD AVOID DENTAL INJURIES?

As children start moving around and exploring more actively around the age of two, they may become more prone to accidents and injuries. To prevent such accidents from happening at home, it is important to take steps to child-proof the house. For older children who engage in sports activities, there is a higher risk of dental trauma. To reduce the likelihood of such injuries, wearing a mouth guard is strongly advised. Additionally, if a child has any teeth alignment issues, it is important to address them as protruding teeth are more vulnerable to injuries during falls or accidents. In such cases, a referral to an orthodontist for further evaluation and treatment may be necessary.

HOW CAN I HELP MY CHILD AVOID GUM DISEASE?

The best way to maintain good oral hygiene while wearing braces is to spend additional time brushing and flossing and to use specific dental products. Food can easily accumulate around the brackets and wires, which, if left for an extended period, can lead to cavities and gum problems. For effective cleaning, I highly recommend using an electric toothbrush since studies have shown that it can remove plaque more efficiently than a manual toothbrush. Spend extra time brushing and use special dental floss that can fit between the wires and teeth.

If oral hygiene is not optimal, it will be helpful to use a prescribed toothpaste with added fluoride. Another useful product is MI Paste, which can prevent demineralization, the white spots that typically develop underneath the brackets, especially in patients with poor oral hygiene. Follow your dental provider instructions and attend regular check-ups to ensure that your braces are correctly maintained and your teeth remain healthy.

HOW CAN I HELP MY CHILD MAINTAIN GOOD ORAL HYGIENE WHILE WEARING BRACES?

When you have braces, it's important to take extra care of your teeth and gums. I recommend using an electric toothbrush to brush your teeth in the morning and at night. With braces, there is a higher risk of food getting stuck around the brackets and wires, so it's important to brush thoroughly. You should also use special dental floss that can fit in between the wires and teeth, and consider using other products that contain fluoride to strengthen your teeth. Another helpful product is MI Paste, which can help with remineralization and prevent the start of cavities. Remember to follow your orthodontist's instructions and attend regular check-ups to ensure that your braces are properly maintained and your teeth stay healthy.

HOW CAN I HELP MY CHILD AVOID TOOTH SENSITIVITY?

When dental enamel wears down, it can lead to tooth sensitivity. This can be caused by grinding or dental erosion, which wears away the enamel over time. To address these issues, it is important to identify the underlying causes. Teeth grinding can be managed with a mouthguard or other dental appliances, while dental erosion can be prevented by avoiding highly acidic foods and drinks.

The best approach to sensitivity depends on its severity. For mild cases, using products like MI Paste can help mineralize the tooth structure and strengthen the teeth. For more severe cases, a filling may be necessary to address tooth wear. In some instances, a combination of these solutions may be recommended based on the individual case.

6.5 - DENTAL WORK

by Dr. AURORA ALVA FROM GERMANY 🏴

WHAT ARE THE MOST COMMON DENTAL PROBLEMS IN CHILDREN?

The most common dental problem in children is cavities, which are often caused by a combination of poor oral hygiene and frequent high sugar consumption. To decrease the risk of getting cavities, it is important to brush properly and regularly and limit the frequency of sugar intake, especially outside of mealtimes.

WHAT CAN I DO IF MY CHILD HAS A DENTAL EMERGENCY?

To address any dental emergencies, it is recommended to schedule a consultation with a dentist. During the consultation, the dentist will examine the affected tooth and may take an X-ray to assess the issue. Based on the findings, further treatment options can be discussed. If a dentist is not available, take your child to the emergency room. Teledentistry is also an option for emergency consultations.

IS IT NECESSARY FOR MY CHILD TO HAVE DENTAL X-RAYS TAKEN?

Whether your child needs X-rays at the dentist will depend on various factors such as age, risk of cavities, and emergency situations like tooth trauma or cavity pain. X-rays help the dentist assess your child's teeth and development. Generally, X-rays are recommended when the back teeth come into contact around age four.

215

Depending on the dentist's assessment, X-rays can be taken of individual teeth or both sides of the mouth. By age six, a panoramic X-ray is usually recommended. This type of X-ray allows the dentist to see all growing teeth, both baby and adult ones, as well as the jaws. If your child has good oral hygiene and no cavities, X-rays are usually recommended every 24 months. However, if your child has a higher risk for cavities, the dentist may recommend X-rays every six months instead.

WHAT IS THE BEST WAY TO TREAT A CHILD'S CAVITIES?

When deciding how to treat a cavity in a child, various factors must be considered, including the size and number of cavities, parental involvement, age, and the child's level of cooperation. For young children with small cavities that are not causing pain, a conservative approach may be recommended. For example, monitoring the cavities and making changes at home to improve oral hygiene and eliminate juice and milk intake outside of mealtimes.

Silver diamine fluoride (SDF) may also be recommended as a cavity-arresting solution that involves no drilling and requires only a small amount of liquid to be applied to the cavity. For larger cavities that cause pain, more extensive treatments such as drilling or spoon excavator removal may be necessary. These procedures are usually followed by filling or a crown. The dentist should be consulted to discuss the best course of action for each individual case.

WHAT IS DENTAL SEALANT, AND IS IT NECESSARY FOR MY CHILD?

Back teeth usually have deep grooves and fissures on their chewing surfaces, which makes it easy for food to accumulate and harder for the toothbrush to remove all the food. Sealants are used to "seal" the chewing surfaces of baby and permanent back teeth to prevent the development of cavities. Recommending sealants depends on the patient's oral hygiene and the anatomy of the teeth.

WHAT ARE THE BENEFITS OF ORTHODONTIC TREATMENT FOR CHILDREN?

Orthodontic treatment in children offers several benefits, with the main advantage being the early identification and treatment of orthodontic issues while the child's jaw and teeth are still developing. This allows for more effective and efficient treatment, which may result in a reduced need for orthodontic intervention in the future.

Correcting dental issues such as crowding, crooked teeth, or bite issues at an early age can have an impact on a child's oral hygiene, speech development, and self-esteem. It is recommended that children receive an orthodontic evaluation by the age of seven to assess their dental development and identify any potential issues that may require early orthodontic intervention.

IS IT OKAY FOR MY CHILD TO PLAY SPORTS WITH BRACES?

When participating in rough sports or activities, it is highly advisable to wear a sports guard specially designed to protect the teeth from potential injuries, especially if the teeth protrude. Consulting a dental provider is crucial in determining the appropriate sports guard to use while wearing braces.

WHAT ARE THE RISKS OF NOT TREATING MY CHILD'S CAVITIES?

I usually offer parents different treatment options for treating cavities, and I openly discuss the benefits and risks of each of them, including the risks of not treating a cavity. I give my recommendation of what I would think to be the best treatment option, but I ultimately have the parent make the decision. Risks of untreated cavities can range from pain, difficulty eating, speech issues, and behavioral problems. I try to emphasize to parents the main concern, which is a child living in pain and the impact pain has on their quality of life.

HOW CAN I PREVENT BABY BOTTLE TOOTH DECAY IN MY CHILD?

Baby bottle tooth decay, also known as early childhood caries, is a common dental issue that can be prevented by taking a few simple steps. The first step is to establish a dental home for your child by the age of 6 months, where you can receive guidance from a dentist on how to prevent tooth decay. This guidance includes instructions on oral hygiene, such as brushing your child's teeth with a smear of toothpaste from the age of 6 months to 3 years, and diet, such as establishing a feeding schedule, limiting juice intake, and avoiding putting the child to sleep with milk beyond 12 months.

HOW CAN I FIND A PAEDIATRIC DENTIST FOR MY CHILD?

The American Academy of Pediatric Dentistry website is the best resource for finding a dentist in your area. You can find a list of pediatric dentists by entering your zip code.

HOW CAN I HELP MY CHILD MAINTAIN GOOD ORAL HYGIENE WHILE WEARING APPLIANCES?

When wearing orthodontic appliances or space maintainers it is important to avoid sticky foods as they can easily get trapped on the appliances or space maintainers. Thorough toothbrushing and flossing are essential, with special attention paid to the back teeth and checking for food accumulation around the appliance or space maintainer bands. Additionally, MI paste can be used to protect teeth from demineralization. This paste contains calcium, phosphate, and fluoride, which can help prevent decalcification around the brackets or bands. It is important to follow your dentist's instructions for using MI paste properly.

6.6 - FEAR/PAIN

by Dr. AURORA ALVA FROM GERMANY

IS SEDATION DENTISTRY NECESSARY FOR CHILDREN?

To achieve successful dental outcomes, sedation is sometimes necessary for children who are too scared or unable to remain still during treatment. Laughing gas is a mild sedation option, while oral sedation medications or general anesthesia offer higher levels of sedation. It is important to evaluate a child's medical history and overall health before proceeding with any sedation method due to the risks associated with them.

For example, laughing gas can increase the risk of vomiting and aspiration, while some oral sedation medications can cause respiratory issues. Anatomical factors like the size of a child's tonsils or tongue can also interfere with their airways during deep sedation. Therefore, sedation is only recommended after careful evaluation and consideration of a child's dental and medical condition, as well as the risks and benefits. For very young children, I would offer conservative treatment alternatives over sedation, such as silver diamine fluoride.

This approach can help avoid the risks associated with sedation and offer a less invasive option for dental treatment. Silver diamine fluoride is a liquid that can arrest cavities and can be applied easily without the need for sedation or general anesthesia. It is important to note that every child's dental needs are different, and a thorough evaluation is necessary to determine the most appropriate treatment plan.

HOW CAN I HELP MY CHILD COPE WITH TOOTH LOSS?

The loss of a child's tooth due to cavities or natural causes can be an opportunity to educate them on dental health. We can use this moment to teach them about the importance of good oral hygiene and the consequences of unhealthy habits such as excessive sugar consumption or lack of brushing. It is important to acknowledge that these behaviors contributed to the problem, but also to reassure them that changes can be made to prevent it from happening again. We can explain that losing baby teeth is a natural part of growing up and that a new, permanent tooth will eventually replace it.

HOW CAN I RELIEVE MY CHILD'S TOOTH ERUPTION PAIN?

There are a few approaches I may recommend for teething discomfort. Massaging the gums or having the child bite on teething rings can help. In extreme cases, pain medications may be necessary. However, I would caution against using pain relief oral gels, especially in children under two years of age, due to the risks associated with developing a potentially fatal condition called methemoglobinemia.

WHAT ARE THE RISKS OF USING TEETHING GELS AND CREAMS?

Teething gels or creams containing benzocaine pose a significant risk of methemoglobinemia, a potentially fatal blood disorder. Due to this serious condition, benzocaine-containing products are contraindicated for children under two years of age. In general, I do not recommend using teething gels or creams on children.

HOW CAN I HELP MY CHILD RECOVER AFTER A DENTAL PROCEDURE?

Following a child's dental treatment, two concerns often arise: lip biting due to numbness and discomfort after the numbing wears off. It is essential to reassure children that numbness is only temporary and encourage parents to observe them to prevent accidental lip, tongue, or cheek biting. We recommend a soft diet until the numbing medication wears off, and if the procedure was extensive or involved multiple teeth extractions, pain medication may be given before the numbing medication wears off. Additionally, for longer procedures, we suggest that children rest for the remainder of the day, follow a soft diet, and watch their favorite movie.

6.7 - MONEY

by Dr. AURORA ALVA FROM GERMANY 🇩🇪

WHAT IS THE COST OF PAEDIATRIC DENTAL CARE?

The restorative dental treatments for children and adults share some similarities. The cost for fillings is relatively equal, but for more complex treatments such as crowns or root canals, the cost for adults is typically higher. Additionally, insurance may not cover sedation for children, while adults usually do not require sedation unless medically necessary.

ARE THOSE COVERED BY THE GOVERNMENT?

Most child dental procedures in the USA are typically covered by the government. However, coverage may vary across states, and some treatments may not be fully covered. For instance, in Georgia, while silver crowns for back teeth are covered by the government, white zirconia crowns are not. Nonetheless, there is good news, as the state of Georgia has recently started covering the use of silver diamine fluoride.

ARE INSURANCE COVERING CHILD DENTAL CARE?

In the US, specifically in Georgia, government insurance covers laughing gas or nitrous oxide until a certain age, while in Germany, it is considered an out-of-pocket expense. In general, both governments and insurance companies in both countries provide coverage for most necessary dental care for children, although there may be some exceptions.

6.8 - HABITS

by Dr. AURORA ALVA FROM GERMANY

IS THUMB-SUCKING HARMFUL TO MY CHILD'S TEETH?

If a child continues the habit of thumb-sucking beyond 36 months, there is a risk of developing an open bite and posterior crossbites. These changes are usually caused by the force applied to the teeth and jaws during thumb sucking, and the effects can be permanent depending on the age and frequency of the habit. It is important to consult with a pediatric dentist for evaluation and treatment, especially if your child is three years of age or older.

HOW CAN I ENCOURAGE MY CHILD TO STOP THUMB-SUCKING?

There are several methods to help stop the habit, such as using a calendar to track progress, applying nail-biting medication to the fingers, using a special glove as a reminder, or using an orthodontic appliance as a last resort. It is important to prepare the child for these treatments in advance to avoid any negative associations with them.

HOW CAN I PREVENT MY CHILD FROM GRINDING THEIR TEETH AT NIGHT?

Teeth grinding in children has been linked to various causes. Fortunately, unlike adults, children who grind their teeth usually outgrow the habit. As dentists, we can identify signs of teeth grinding by visually examining the teeth and observing wear patterns. Treatment options may involve using a custom mouthguard to protect the teeth or addressing underlying issues like emotional stress.

WHAT ARE THE DANGERS OF SHARING UTENSILS AND DRINKS WITH MY CHILD?

Several studies have shown that mothers can transmit their own oral bacteria to their children through activities like sharing utensils. However, this transmission does not necessarily pose a significant danger to the child's oral health. Instead, the mother's own oral hygiene habits and behaviors have a greater influence on the child's risk for developing cavities. For example, if the mother practices good oral hygiene, she is more likely to encourage the same habits in her children.

HOW CAN I HELP MY CHILD AVOID JAW PROBLEMS?

To prevent future jaw problems, it is important to prioritize prevention and early detection. I recommend consulting with a specialist in cases of orthodontic issues or problems related to the temporomandibular joint (TMJ). Your pediatric dentist can provide referrals to either an orthodontist or TMJ specialist. It is important to address TMJ disorders early as they are complex and can worsen over time.

HOW CAN I PREVENT DENTAL PROBLEMS IN MY CHILD WHILE THEY ARE SLEEPING?

Preventing dental problems during sleep involves two main issues, the development of cavities and bruxism. To prevent cavities, it is important for children to go to bed with clean teeth. At night, saliva production decreases, which increases the risk of caries developing. Regarding bruxism, addressing the cause is the first step. If the child has all their adult teeth, a mouthguard may be recommended to prevent damage to the teeth and jaw.

This is **ALPHA DENTISTRY vol. 3, PAEDIATRIC DENTISTRY FAQ**. Welcome to the Alphas.

Dr. BAK NGUYEN

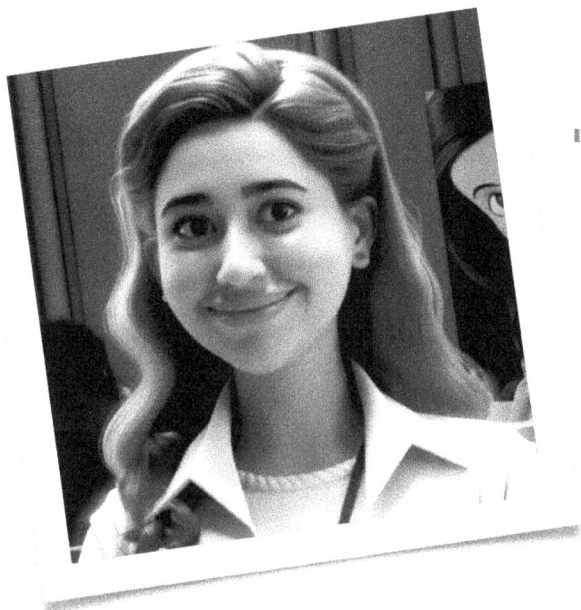

Dr. NOUR AMMAR,
DMD, MS

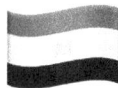

From EGYPT , **Dr. NOUR AMMAR**, BDS, MS. She is a dedicated specialist in pediatric dentistry and dental public health hailing from Egypt. With an impressive educational background from Alexandria University's Faculty of Dentistry, including graduating top of her class in her bachelor's degree and master's degree, Dr. Ammar has already achieved so much in her field. She has served as a teaching assistant at the same institution for five years, demonstrating her passion for sharing knowledge with others. In addition to her academic accomplishments, Dr. Ammar is also a Harvard alumnus and has participated in a clinical research program there. Her clinical work has earned her several distinguished prizes and awards, demonstrating her exceptional skills and commitment to improving patient outcomes. Currently pursuing a Ph.D. at the University of Munich (LMU) in Germany, Dr. Ammar is committed to raising awareness and knowledge of oral health, particularly among parents and children. Her vision of improving access to dental care for underprivileged or remote populations is being realized through the development of an AI program that can assist primary healthcare centers in identifying different dental pathologies without the real-time presence of a specialist. With her passion for pediatric dentistry and dental public health, Dr. Nour Ammar is a true asset to her profession.

Dr. Nour Ammar was introduced by our common friend, Dr. Aurora Alva. I learnt to know Dr. Nour right on the field, as we were collaborating and brainstorming for this book. A brilliant mind, a kind heart, and a doctor with vision is how Dr. Ammar struck me. Yes, I had the objective to complete this book, but very quickly, it became very tempting to derail the conversation to artificial intelligence and how Dr. Nour and her team are looking to implement it to improve care accessibility in remote areas.

Dr. Nour is a Ph.D. candidate at the time of this writing. Exchanging with her, I have great hope for the future leadership of our profession. Not only because of her kindness and professionalism but also for her drive and willingness to make a difference.

This is a mere beginning, Dr. Nour. Please join me in welcoming Dr. Nour Ammar into the Alphas.

This is **ALPHA DENTISTRY vol. 3, PAEDIATRIC DENTISTRY FAQ**. Welcome to the Alphas.

Dr. BAK NGUYEN

CHAPTER 7
"PAEDIATRIC DENTISTRY"
by Dr. NOUR AMMAR

FROM EGYPT

7.1 - DEFINITIONS

by Dr. NOUR AMMAR FROM EGYPT ⬰

WHAT IS THE BEST TYPE OF TOOTHBRUSH FOR MY CHILD?

Generally, any small-size soft bristle toothbrush would be fine. When selecting a toothbrush for children, it is important to choose a small size toothbrush that can reach behind the molars, both upper and lower, and on the lingual (tongue facing) and facial (cheek/lip facing) sides. Using a brush that is too large can cause an aggravated gag reflex or make the process unpleasant for the child.

WHAT IS THE ROLE OF FLUORIDE IN PREVENTING CAVITIES?

Fluoride is a mineral that helps combat dental caries. It has been scientifically proven to be one of the most effective and inexpensive ways to prevent caries in children. If your children use a fluoridated water source as their primary source of water intake, then there is a great chance that fluoride is reaching their teeth. Naturally, the concentration and availability will vary depending on your location. Fluoride makes enamel (outer hard layer of the tooth crown) more resistant to the corrosive action of acids that are produced by oral bacteria. This in turn slows the decay process. In fact, several studies have concluded that fluoride can even stop the progression of dental decay that has already begun!

WHAT IS THE DIFFERENCE BETWEEN A PAEDIATRIC DENTIST AND A GENERAL DENTIST?

Although all dentists are trained in general dentistry, paediatric dentists undergo additional specialized education in treating children, including clinical and didactic training that intensively focuses on the paediatric patient. As a result, they develop greater expertise in preventing and treating dental diseases in children, usually between the ages of zero and twelve. Furthermore, they are better trained to advise and educate parents on how to safeguard their children's oral health during the critical time of transitioning from baby to adult teeth.

While a general dentist may provide dental care to children, a paediatric dentist is fully equipped to handle the wide spectrum of children's behaviour, as well as any special conditions or concerns that may arise. Orthodontics is a separate speciality from paediatric dentistry, and while orthodontists may address certain dental issues related to tooth alignment, paediatric dentists are focused on the prevention and maintenance of the oral health of children from the time of their first tooth.

WHAT ARE THE MOST COMMON ORTHODONTIC PROBLEMS IN CHILDREN?

One common issue that parents report is that their child has two rows of teeth in the lower jaw, which is commonly referred to as 'shark teeth'. This happens when the permanent tooth grows behind the primary one, causing crowding in the lower front teeth area. If the child is within the normal range of the tooth eruption schedule, which is typically around six years of age with a six-month variation, I would advise parents to wait and see for two to three more months. If the primary tooth becomes more mobile during this time, then it is on its way to natural shedding. If not, a simple and painless extraction of the primary teeth can be performed, which usually resolves the issue by allowing the permanent teeth to shift to place.

HOW CAN I TELL IF MY CHILD NEEDS ORTHODONTIC TREATMENT?

It is recommended that the child completes a biannual dental check-up with their paediatric dentist. Paediatric dentists are well-versed in the normal sequence of eruption and shedding of primary and permanent dentition and can tell you if there's something wrong going on. If your child needs orthodontic treatment, your dentist or pediatric dentist will refer you to an orthodontist for specialized treatment. So, make sure to keep up with regular dental check-ups and don't hesitate to ask your dentist any questions you may have about your child's dental health.

WHAT ARE THE BENEFITS OF DENTAL SEALANTS FOR CHILDREN?

Sealants are an effective way to prevent decay and cavities from forming on the chewing surfaces of your child's molar teeth. These surfaces are often irregular with grooves and valleys that can trap food and bacteria, making them difficult to clean. Sealants can fill these grooves and create a smoother surface that is easier to clean and can protect teeth for a long period of time. Keep in mind that sealants need to be followed up and reapplied periodically. The success depends on the proper application technique and regular checkups to ensure that they are not damaged or leaking.

7.2 - PREVENTION

by Dr. NOUR AMMAR FROM EGYPT

HOW CAN I PREPARE MY CHILD FOR THEIR FIRST DENTAL VISIT?
There are several things to consider. Firstly, I would like to emphasize the depth of parental influence on a child's attitude toward dental visits. Children often emulate their parents' thoughts, opinions, and anxiety about visits to the dentist. It is important to realize the power of positivity and encouragement when discussing dental visits with children. Parents should be mindful of their words and facial expressions and try to explain things simply and optimistically.

Additionally, it can be helpful for dental care to have videos or pictures available online that introduce the practice and its staff to children. Another suggestion is to offer young patients a non-operative visit during off-hours, allowing them to familiarize themselves with the office and the people who work there. These efforts can help make dental care a regular and accepted part of a child's life and contribute to the establishment of what we call a dental home.

HOW CAN I HELP MY CHILD OVERCOME THEIR FEAR OF THE DENTIST?
When it comes to children who have no previous dental experience, it is important to take some steps to help them feel comfortable and confident before their first appointment. One way to do this is to bring them in for a visit beforehand, where they can casually meet their

dentist, see the office, and get a feel for what the experience will be like. You can also show them pictures or videos of other children or adults who have had calm and positive experiences at the dentist to help them understand that it can be a pain-free experience.

As a parent, it is important to talk positively about dental visits and let your child know that you are there to support them throughout the process. Although medical decisions are ultimately in the hands of the parent, it can be empowering for the child to know that their concerns and fears will be heard and addressed. Furthermore, pediatric dentists are trained to use an array of behavior management techniques to help successfully navigate a child's dental experience.

Consider allowing your child to bring a favorite stuffed animal, toy, or blanket to their appointment. This can provide them with a sense of comfort and familiarity. Lastly, accompany your child to their dental appointment and stay with them throughout the visit if possible. This will help them feel safe and supported and can also help ease any anxiety they may be feeling. Overall, taking the time to prepare your child for their first dental visit can help establish a positive and lifelong relationship with dental care.

HOW CAN I PREPARE MY CHILD FOR A DENTAL PROCEDURE?

It's important to approach the topic of visiting the dentist positively and explain to your child that it is a necessary part of maintaining good dental and overall health. You can ease their fears by asking the dentist for a tour of the clinic and introducing them to the staff. This will help them become familiar with the environment and feel more comfortable during their appointments.

IS IT OKAY FOR CHILDREN TO CONSUME SUGARY FOODS AND DRINKS?

It's important to maintain a balance when it comes to your child's diet. While we don't want to completely deprive children of sweets and sugary drinks, it's important to practice moderation. I have two concerns about excessive sugar intake, nutrition, and oral hygiene. From a dental perspective, it's best to have sugary treats immediately after a meal to limit the time that the sugars stay in contact with the teeth. This is essential because sugar is a culprit in fuelling acid-producing bacteria in the mouth, leading to tooth decay.

As for preventing damage before it happens, paediatric dentists offer a dietary analysis service to parents who are interested in getting more specific information about their child's diet. You can ask for a diet analysis for your child. You will be asked to precisely record all your child's meals and snacks, including the specific foods and times for at least one day. Your provider will then analyze the patterns and let you know if your child is consuming too much or too frequent sugar throughout the day, and how to make adjustments if necessary.

After all, there is a direct link between dental decay and obesity. As a dentist, I care about the overall health and well-being of my patients and their families. But in the case of severe diet discrepancies, I can refer you to other medical specialities more suited to support your child's nutrition.

CAN MY CHILD STILL ENJOY SWEET TREATS WHILE MAINTAINING GOOD ORAL HYGIENE?

Firstly, it's important to note that sugary snacks and drinks should be consumed in moderation, and not as a frequent indulgence. Secondly, brushing the teeth or rinsing the mouth with water after consuming sugary items is a good step, but it's also important to wait at least 10 minutes after eating before brushing, as brushing immediately after can damage the tooth enamel. In summary, limit the consumption of sugary snacks and drinks to occasional treats and ensure that your child practises proper oral hygiene measures.

HOW CAN I ENSURE THAT MY CHILD IS RECEIVING ADEQUATE NUTRITION FOR HEALTHY TEETH?

While there is no specific nutrition required for teeth development, it is important to ensure that your child is receiving a healthy and well-balanced diet that meets their overall nutritional needs as recommended by your paediatrician. This would include a wide range of vegetables, fruits, grains, dairy products, protein, and healthy. Nowadays, paediatric dentists are engaged in nutrition education. If your dentist believes that your child is suffering from malnutrition, they can support him by referring you to the necessary nutritional counseling from a paediatrician or nutritional specialist. By maintaining good communication with your dentist and staying vigilant about your child's dental health, you can help prevent future problems.

HOW CAN I ENSURE MY CHILD IS GETTING ENOUGH FLUORIDE?

This is an important question that depends on various factors such as your location and the dietary habits of your child. Therefore, it's difficult to give a general answer without a specific analysis and further information provided to your dentist. Age, location, diet, and physical needs can all play a role in determining the appropriate fluoride intake for your child. It's important to distinguish between fluoride as a systematic supplement versus an oral or topical supplement. Fluoride deficiency is rare, so consuming fluoridated water and brushing teeth twice a day with fluoridated toothpaste is usually sufficient for topical fluoride supplementation. Systematic fluoride supplementation is generally not needed.

HOW CAN I PREVENT ORTHODONTIC PROBLEMS IN MY CHILD?

Preventing orthodontic abnormalities is a complex issue, but there are some things that parents can do to help reduce the risk. An important step is to ensure that your child maintains good oral hygiene and avoids severe tooth decay, as it can cause teeth to shift and become misaligned. Additionally, it's important to monitor your child for any oral habits such as thumb sucking, tongue thrusting, or mouth breathing, as these habits can also contribute to orthodontic problems, especially in the mixed dentition stage when the baby teeth are shedding and the permanent teeth erupting.

This is a time when children are most prone to developing orthodontic problems, so it is crucial to keep an eye out for any abnormalities and avoid any habits. If you notice any of these habits, it's important to talk to your child's dentist or orthodontist for advice on possible early interventions.

7.3 - TIME

by Dr. NOUR AMMAR FROM EGYPT

WHAT IS THE BEST AGE FOR A CHILD TO START SEEING A DENTIST?

We recommend that children complete their first dental visit by their first birthday or when their teeth start to erupt, typically around six months of age. The first dental visit should take place when you notice the two lower central front teeth coming in.

HOW OFTEN SHOULD MY CHILD SEE A DENTIST?

The frequency of dental checkups for your child can vary depending on their risk of developing dental problems. Typically, low-risk children should go every six months, while high-risk children may be asked to come every three months. Factors that can increase risk include inconsistent oral hygiene, existing dental caries, frequent consumption of sugary foods, and poor nutrition. Your dentist will let you know when your child's next checkup would be.

WHAT IS THE BEST AGE FOR A CHILD TO GET ORTHODONTIC TREATMENT?

OK, this is a complex matter and depends on the specific orthodontic issue your child has. Some problems can be treated as early as six years of age, while others require waiting until all permanent teeth have erupted, which usually occurs around twelve years of age. Your dentist will be able to determine the best course of action based on your child's individual needs after completing the needed investigations. If a complex problem is at hand, your dentist will guide you toward the necessary treatment, which may involve seeing an orthodontic specialist. That being said, paediatric dentists are trained to perform removable orthodontic treatments, so it may not always be necessary to see an orthodontist.

WHAT ARE THE SIGNS OF TEETH ERUPTION IN A CHILD?
It's common for children to be fussy and irritable when their teeth are erupting. They may also have slightly higher temperatures and produce more saliva. You may notice they are not interested in their usual activities or play. If you check inside their mouth, you'll see a discolored tender spot where the tooth is expected to erupt. Over-the-counter gels or ointments can be used up to twice a day to provide relief, but you can also try anything cool like chewing on frozen fruits. Typically, this discomfort lasts for about two weeks until the tooth emerges and resolves spontaneously.

7.4 - MAINTENANCE

by Dr. NOUR AMMAR FROM EGYPT

WHAT IS THE RIGHT WAY TO CLEAN MY CHILD'S TEETH?
Maintaining your child's oral hygiene should begin very early. By the time your child shows signs of the eruption of their first tooth, an oral hygiene regimen must be in place. Parents are advised to supervise and help their children clean their teeth. Children up to the age of six

or seven may not clean their teeth efficiently or correctly, so parents should supervise them and intervene when needed. Use a small soft toothbrush and a brush in a horizontal motion on all the sides of the teeth. On the side facing the cheeks, the side inside, and the side that is chewed on, on the lower and upper rows of teeth.

HOW CAN I ENCOURAGE MY CHILD TO BRUSH THEIR TEETH REGULARLY?

Encouraging children to brush their teeth regularly requires incorporating it into their daily routine, such as during bedtime or morning routines. It's useful to set a consistent schedule for brushing and to make it a group activity, such as brushing teeth together with parents. Brushing should last approximately two minutes, and parents can use songs or timers as indicators to help children know when to stop brushing. This will help children form healthy habits and maintain good oral hygiene. In addition, it is beneficial to talk to your child about the importance of having a clean mouth and healthy teeth and that it is an essential part of personal care.

HOW CAN I PREVENT TOOTH DECAY IN MY CHILD'S BABY TEETH?

There are several things you can do to help your child maintain good dental health which all begin with setting an appropriate oral hygiene practice in place. For children who have no erupted teeth yet, use a gauze or silicone finger toothbrush to massage their gums after feedings. As for children under 3 years of age, a rice-sized amount of fluoridated children's toothpaste should be used with a small brush twice daily. While in children aged 3 to 6, a pea-sized amount of toothpaste should be used. Limit your child's intake of sugary foods to no more than twice a day to control bacterial growth in the mouth. Dental caries, or tooth decay, is generally not reversible, but the very early stages can be treated with brushing, fluoride treatment, or a change in diet.

HOW CAN I PREVENT MY CHILD FROM DEVELOPING DENTAL ANXIETY?

Dental anxiety is a common issue among children. Firstly, start early by introducing your child to dental care as soon as their first tooth appears. This will help them get used to the idea of dental visits and make it a routine part of their life. Secondly, use positive language when discussing dental care with your child. Avoid using words that may cause fear or anxiety, such as "pain" or "hurt." Instead, emphasize the benefits of good oral health and make dental care a positive experience. Thirdly, you can play pretend dentist with your child to help them get comfortable with the experience.

Let them "check" your teeth, and then you can "check" theirs. This can help them familiarise themselves with the dental visit process and make it less scary. A good paediatric dentist should be able to put your child at ease and make the visit pleasant. By following these tips, you can help prevent your child from developing dental anxiety and create a positive dental experience for them.

HOW CAN I HELP MY CHILD AVOID DENTAL INJURIES?

There are several things to keep in mind when it comes to your child's dental safety. Firstly, it's important to supervise all children, but especially those under the age of three as they may be prone to falls and accidents at home. Older children should be made aware of the importance of dental hygiene and the risks associated with damaging their teeth. Encourage them not to bite hard objects or eat things that shouldn't be eaten. And if your child has any crooked or misaligned teeth, consider talking to your dentist about orthodontic treatment to straighten them and reduce the risk of injury.

For children who play contact sports, a custom-fit dental guard is recommended. Although over-the-counter guards are available, they may not fit as well and can cause irritation or injuries to the dental soft tissues. Custom-fit guards, which are made from impressions of your child's teeth, are more comfortable and have a longer lifespan.

HOW CAN I HELP MY CHILD AVOID GUM DISEASE?
Preventing cavities is important because cavities and gum disease are interconnected. Cavities can lead to the proliferation of bacteria that can also affect the gums. Therefore, if you prevent cavities, you can prevent gum disease. Children with a lot of cavities or broken teeth often have inflamed, tender, or painful gums. It is also important to note that some children have a habit of sticking objects into their mouths, which can cause injury and pain, and may require complex treatments. Ultimately, educate your child on the signs of gum disease such as red, swollen, or bleeding gums, and encourage them to report any symptoms to you or their dentist immediately.

HOW CAN I HELP MY CHILD MAINTAIN GOOD ORAL HYGIENE WHILE WEARING BRACES?
It's crucial to emphasize that children with braces or intraoral appliances are at a higher risk of developing

dental caries. To combat this, it's important to use a toothbrush specifically designed to clean braces which has extra-long bristles that extend beyond the brackets and wires. Additionally, it's essential to take excellent care of oral hygiene, especially after eating, by actively rinsing the mouth and removing any food particles that may be trapped in the wires or attachments if teeth brushing is not possible at the moment. It's also advised to avoid consuming sticky foods or candies that can easily break the braces or become lodged within the braces' components.

HOW CAN I HELP MY CHILD AVOID TOOTH SENSITIVJTY?

Sensitivity in children is not a common occurrence, it may arise in association with certain pathologies, diseases, or syndromes. If your child suffers from dental sensitivity, you can help alleviate the discomfort by using desensitizing toothpaste, which can close the pores on the tooth surface that may be sensitive to external stimulation. Limit consumption of acidic foods and drinks (citrus fruits, soda, and sports drinks) that can erode tooth enamel, which can aggravate tooth sensitivity.

However, dental treatments are available in clinics to address sensitivity problems. If your child is complaining about sensitivity to anything hot or cold, you should be concerned because it is a sign of caries or tooth pulp inflammation. The tooth pulp is a living system with vessels and blood inside. Sensitivity indicates an abnormality or inflammation of some sort. Furthermore, if your child experiences pain when biting on a tooth, it could be indicative of gum disease inflammation.

7.5 - DENTAL WORK

by Dr. NOUR AMMAR FROM EGYPT

WHAT ARE THE MOST COMMON DENTAL PROBLEMS IN CHILDREN?

Without a doubt, the most common dental problem in children is dental caries, especially in primary teeth. It can have many negative consequences. It's essential to keep an eye out for signs of decay and visit the dentist twice a year.

WHAT CAN I DO IF MY CHILD HAS A DENTAL EMERGENCY?

Addressing dental emergencies as soon as possible is of paramount importance ensuring good treatment outcomes for your child's injury. It is recommended to contact your child's regular dentist first, but if they are not available, seek the nearest available dentist regardless of their specialty or if you've visited them before. Most dentists prioritize emergency cases and will provide prompt treatment. If your child has a knocked-out permanent tooth, try to gently reinsert it into its socket after gently rinsing it with lukewarm water.

Avoid touching the tooth's root or holding it from that part as it will severely decrease the chances of tooth survival. Furthermore, if a baby tooth is knocked out, do not attempt to put it back in its socket, this should only be done with permanent teeth. If that's not possible, keep the tooth moist by placing it in milk or saliva and see a dentist as soon as possible.

IS IT NECESSARY FOR MY CHILD TO HAVE DENTAL X-RAYS TAKEN?

There are specific guidelines for the type and frequency of X-rays that children need. Generally, routine or follow-up dental X-rays are taken starting at six years of age. Pediatric dentists are trained to limit the amount of possible radiation that the children are exposed to. If your child has a low risk of developing dental problems and is not experiencing any issues, X-rays may only be needed once a year. However, if there are signs of inflammation or cavities, the frequency may be increased to twice a year, and specific X-rays may be needed for problem areas. Dental X-rays are low-risk procedures and your dentist will determine the appropriate frequency based on your child's condition.

WHAT IS THE BEST WAY TO TREAT A CHILD'S CAVITIES?

Great question! It's important to know that the choice of treatment for a cavity will depend on several factors, such as the type of tooth, size and severity of the cavity, if there are any special considerations, and the patient's and their parent's preferences. Your dentist will assess the condition and discuss the options with you, including the benefits and risks of each. Amalgam and composite are two common filling materials used to restore decayed teeth. Amalgam is a silver material that has been used for decades, while composite is a tooth-colored resin that can blend in with natural tooth color. Both have their advantages and disadvantages, and your dentist can explain these to you in detail.

On the other hand, a crown may be recommended for more extensive decay or damage to the tooth. A crown is a protective cap that covers the entire tooth, and it can be made from different materials, such as metal (silver-colored) or zirconia (tooth colored). Your dentist may recommend a crown if a filling will not be sufficient to restore the tooth's function and appearance, or will not provide ideal treatment outcomes. Ultimately, the decision should be made with the advice of your dentist while taking into account your preferences and the best treatment option for the specific case of your child.

WHAT IS DENTAL SEALANT, AND IS IT NECESSARY FOR MY CHILD?

Sealants are an effective way to prevent decay and cavities from forming on the chewing surfaces of your child's molars. These surfaces are often irregular with grooves and valleys that can trap food and bacteria, making them difficult to clean. Being a thin liquid material, it can be applied to fill in these grooves and create a smoother surface that is easier to clean and can protect teeth for a length of time. Applying sealants effectively helps to prevent the initiation of cavities. However, not all children are good candidates for sealants, as it depends on the specific condition of their teeth. Children with smooth, shallow-cusped teeth may not need sealants, while those with deep grooves and pits may benefit from them.

Your dentist can evaluate your child's teeth and determine if sealants would be a good option for them. Keep in mind that sealants need to be followed up and reapplied periodically. The success depends on the proper application technique and regular checkups to ensure that they are not faulty or leaking.

WHAT ARE THE BENEFITS OF ORTHODONTIC TREATMENT FOR CHILDREN?

As a dentist, we have three main objectives when providing dental treatment: to restore function, to improve aesthetics, and to eliminate or prevent pain. Orthodontic problems can have a significant impact on a child's self-confidence, especially during their school years, when they may experience peer pressure. As a result, orthodontic treatment may be necessary not only to improve dental health but also to positively impact a child's personal development and self-esteem.

In addition to improving aesthetics, it's important to ensure that a child's teeth are aligned correctly to create the best environment possible for their permanent teeth to erupt in their correct places, thus preventing future misalignment problems. Orthodontic problems can also cause pain, so eliminating this discomfort is another important aspect of treatment. Many of these problems in the primary dentition can be easily addressed. Your pediatric dentist can prevent, intercept, or manage these problems as needed.

IS IT OKAY FOR MY CHILD TO PLAY SPORTS WITH BRACES?

It's important to prioritize protecting your child's braces and orthodontic appliances, this usually means avoiding contact sports. Trauma or injury to the teeth can cause them to break or become more susceptible to damage, and it can also harm the soft tissue around them. In the case of a child wearing braces, getting hit in the mouth during a contact sport can aggravate injuries due to the presence of metallic appliances in the mouth.

To mitigate this risk, if your child is playing contact sports, it's important to invest in a custom-fit mouthguard provided by a dentist rather than an over-the-counter one. Over-the-counter mouthguards are not suitable for children with braces due to the complex structure of orthodontic appliances in which malleable materials can get trapped. It's important to prioritize your child's safety and protect their dental health.

WHAT ARE THE RISKS OF NOT TREATING MY CHILD'S CAVITIES?

It's common for people to underestimate the severity of dental decay, but it's important to understand that it's not just a simple issue and that oral health is part of overall health. A cavity means that the affected tooth has undergone changes in its shape and structure which eventually leads to problems with the neighboring teeth as well. Teeth maintain their position through the tight contacts that they have with adjacent and opposing teeth, so when the size, shape, or place of a tooth changes it affects these contacts in a very unhealthy way.

In addition, the dental cavity is an area where bacteria and food particles can become trapped and retained, creating an environment that encourages further decay and infection. This cycle can continue and spread to other teeth, leading to more extensive damage. It's important to take cavities seriously and seek treatment as soon as possible to prevent further complications and avoid the need for complex treatments.

HOW CAN I PREVENT BABY BOTTLE TOOTH DECAY IN MY CHILD?

Baby bottle tooth decay is unfortunately a very common issue. It is referred to as early childhood caries of which a severe type is possible. This condition occurs when children, who are still nursing or breastfeeding, fall asleep with a continuous source of milk/sugary drink in their mouth. This sweetened liquid provides a continuous source of sugar to the oral bacteria, which in turn use this sugar to thrive and produce acids that break down the tooth structure. The upper front teeth are usually the first to be affected, and the decay often extends to the rest of the teeth mainly on the side facing the cheeks. Treatment of this condition is challenging and traumatic for the child. Thus, it's very important to be vigilant about it in newborns and avoid nursing children to sleep. If it is a must, you should only put water in their bedtime nursing bottle.

HOW CAN I FIND A PAEDIATRIC DENTIST FOR MY CHILD?

You can find paediatric dentists near you by checking your local directory or asking a friend for recommendations. When looking for a dentist for your child, you should prioritize finding someone who is not only knowledgeable and formally trained in this profession, but also compassionate and understanding towards children. It's important to find a dentist who is willing to listen to the parents and take their wishes into consideration, while also providing the necessary information and guidance to make informed decisions about their child's dental treatment.

In addition, a dentist who can establish a positive relationship with your child can make a big difference in ensuring their cooperation and compliance with dental care and can prepare them for a healthy lifelong relationship with oral health.

HOW CAN I HELP MY CHILD MAINTAIN GOOD ORAL HYGIENE WHILE WEARING APPLIANCES?

Any intra-oral appliances can significantly increase the risk of tooth decay. You will typically be instructed on how to assist your child in putting on and taking off their appliance correctly if it is removable. However, it is also essential to keep the appliance itself clean. After the child finishes brushing their teeth, they should clean all surfaces of the appliance with the same toothbrush and paste. This will ensure that all surfaces of the appliance are free of food particles that can attract bacteria and promote dental decay. As for braces, emphasis on the importance of toothbrushing after every meal is important and you can find the dedicated toothbrush types for braces. By taking these steps, you can help prevent other oral diseases from developing and keep your child's mouth healthy.

7.6 - FEAR/PAIN

by Dr. NOUR AMMAR FROM EGYPT

IS SEDATION DENTISTRY NECESSARY FOR CHILDREN?

Dentists resort to sedation after trying other behavior management techniques. While sedation may not be highly acceptable for all patients, it may become a necessity to consider. It is important to talk to your dentist about alternative options before reaching the stage where your child needs sedation for dental treatment and whether conscious sedation or general anesthesia operation would be recommended. These treatment approaches are reserved for complex cases requiring extensive dental treatment and highly uncooperative patients who become uncontrollably disruptive during dental procedures.

Regarding the minimum age for sedation, it is largely dependent on the weight of the child as it determines the dosage of the sedative used. Generally, sedation is not used in patients under three years of age. Consult with your dentist to determine the most appropriate approach for your child's specific needs.

HOW CAN I HELP MY CHILD COPE WITH TOOTH LOSS?

For the most suitable answer, I would recommend that you try to turn to references from your culture. The tradition of celebrating a child's tooth loss can often be found in many cultures. For example, in some cultures, children receive a visit from the tooth fairy and a reward for each lost tooth. In others, losing a tooth is considered a chance for a wish to come true, where the child has the opportunity to make a special wish that the parents usually honor. Regardless of the tradition, it's important to make the experience positive and celebratory for the child and educate them on the normal process of tooth shedding and eruption and how it is important to take care of the new adult teeth as they are not replaceable.

HOW CAN I RELIEVE MY CHILD'S TOOTH ERUPTION PAIN?

There are a few things you can do. Firstly, you can offer them something cold to chew on, such as a chilled teething ring or frozen fruit. Furthermore, over-the-counter gels or ointments can be used up to twice a day to provide relief by numbing the area and reducing discomfort. If needed, oral analgesics can also be prescribed.

WHAT ARE THE RISKS OF USING TEETHING GELS AND CREAMS?

There are a variety of over-the-counter products that are safe to use on children from birth. However, there is a risk of misuse when it comes to teething gels, which are meant to soothe gum pain with a local anesthetic. Unfortunately, many parents overuse the gel by using an excessive amount or by applying it too frequently without considering the proper dosage for their child's age and weight.

This can result in various side effects that include allergic reactions, numbness of the throat if swallowed in excess, and in rare cases, more serious health problems can arise such as methemoglobinemia. In methemoglobinemia, oxygen is unable to bind to hemoglobin in the blood, leading to shortness of breath, and fatigue. To avoid these risks, it's important to adhere to the recommended dosage and frequency of use for any teething gel. If you notice any adverse effects, stop using the product immediately and consult with your child's dentist or pediatrician.

HOW CAN I HELP MY CHILD RECOVER AFTER A DENTAL PROCEDURE?

It's important to provide positive reinforcement and praise for their behavior during dental visits. This can help to build positive associations with dental care and encourage them to continue to cooperate in the future. In terms of rewards, it's important to choose something that is not sugary or harmful to their teeth. Instead, consider taking them to a fun activity or buying them a new toy or book.

WHAT IS THE COST OF PAEDIATRIC DENTAL CARE?

The cost of paediatric dental treatment can vary depending on the complexity of the procedure and the type of behavior management techniques used. For instance, if a child requires advanced techniques such as sedation or complex treatments, the cost will be higher than a routine checkup or cleaning. Additionally, if parents choose to have multiple visits for behavior management techniques, this may also add to the cost. It's important to discuss any potential costs with your dentist and insurance provider beforehand to ensure you are fully informed.

ARE THOSE COVERED BY THE GOVERNMENT?

In Egypt, there are different settings. There are a great number of public teaching hospitals that receive government funding, where most paediatric dental treatments are covered by the government for all citizens. There are also private clinics where treatments can be covered by private insurance, or the patient may choose to pay privately.

IS INSURANCE COVERING CHILD DENTAL CARE?

Yes. However, such coverage would require a specific type of dental insurance or added coverage to an existing insurance plan. Fortunately, there are insurance plans that do cover dental care for children.

7.8 - HABITS

by Dr. NOUR AMMAR FROM EGYPT ▰

IS THUMB-SUCKING HARMFUL TO MY CHILD'S TEETH?

Thumb-sucking is one of the most harmful oral habits that can negatively impact your child's dental health. When a child is sucking his thumb or any finger, he/she exerts inward pressure on the lower teeth and outward pressure on the upper teeth. This can result in the upper teeth protruding and the lower teeth leaning backward, which over time can cause the entire lower jaw to shift backward, leading to an unappealing facial profile. Advanced cases may require orthodontic treatment to correct the position of the lower jaw. Thumb-sucking is a common habit among children, but it should be discouraged by the age of three or three and a half to avoid the possibility of long-term damage. Parents should actively intervene and persuade their children to stop this habit before it becomes a serious problem.

HOW CAN I ENCOURAGE MY CHILD TO STOP THUMB-SUCKING?

Thumb sucking will generally only become a problem if this habit continues for an extended time. Most children stop this habit on their own, usually around the age of three. Otherwise, there is a range of treatments available to help a child stop thumb sucking, starting with the least invasive methods. It is important to make the child aware of the habit since they may not be aware of it. Encouraging the whole family to bring attention to the issue is a good start. If this doesn't work, there are intra-oral appliances that can be used.

The simplest one is a wire that attaches to the upper molar and has a ball or rolling element in front of the tongue. This serves as a reminder to the child to not put their thumb in their mouth. If that doesn't work, a more advanced appliance called a palatal crib can be used. This appliance prevents the child from putting their thumb in their mouth by placing small protruding extensions where the child usually places their thumb. It's important to note that thumb sucking is a natural self-soothing mechanism for children, and it's okay until around three years of age. It's not recommended to forcefully stop a child from thumb sucking from birth.

HOW CAN I PREVENT MY CHILD FROM GRINDING THEIR TEETH AT NIGHT?

Bruxism, also known as teeth grinding, is often associated with psychological factors such as stress and anxiety. Therefore, it's advisable to avoid any negative interactions or stressors in the hours leading up to bedtime and create a calm bedtime routine. Furthermore, limiting your child's caffeine consumption (which can be in the form of fizzy drinks) throughout the day would be very helpful. However, one of the often overlooked causes of bruxism is gastrointestinal problems, specifically an oral microbe called H. pylori. If emotional and social factors have been ruled out, it may be worth checking for this infection as it is a common cause of bruxism in children.

WHAT ARE THE DANGERS OF SHARING UTENSILS AND DRINKS WITH MY CHILD?

Children are born with a relatively low bacterial count in their oral cavity, which makes them naturally less susceptible to dental caries. In contrast, adults have abundant amounts of bacteria in their mouths. It's important to delay the introduction of bacteria to a child's oral cavity as much as possible to prevent the development of dental caries later on. Sharing spoons, for instance, can transfer bacteria to the child's mouth, and can cause the spread of germs and other infections.

HOW CAN I HELP MY CHILD AVOID JAW PROBLEMS?
Abnormal oral habits that develop at a young age can lead to various dental problems. Thumb sucking, mouth breathing, and lip biting are some of the common habits that can cause problems. Parents need to closely monitor their child's habits and ensure that they are not engaging in them frequently. Preventing these habits can help prevent future dental problems.

HOW CAN I PREVENT DENTAL PROBLEMS IN MY CHILD WHILE THEY ARE SLEEPING?
One of the most important things to do is to avoid night feeding, whether it's natural or bottle feeding. Another key point to consider is to see if your child is mouth breathing during sleep, as this can be a symptom of underlying airway abnormalities and can cause severe changes in the shape and structure of the oral cavity. Also, look out for bruxism or teeth clenching and seek treatment for this issue before it causes dental problems.

This is **ALPHA DENTISTRY vol. 3, PAEDIATRIC DENTISTRY FAQ**. Welcome to the Alphas.

Dr. BAK NGUYEN

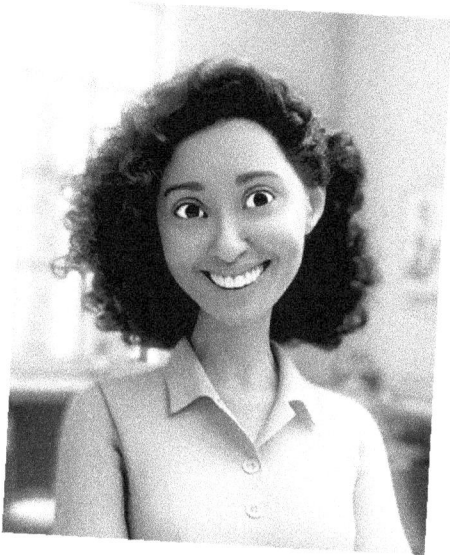

Dr. AILIN CABRERA-MATTA,

DMD, MS, Ph.D.

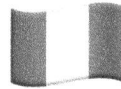

From PERU , **Dr. AILIN CABRERA-MATTA**, DDS, MSc, Ph.D., is an associate professor at the Peruvian University Cayetano Heredia. In addition to being a pediatrician, she holds a master's degree in epidemiology, a master's degree in pediatric dentistry, and a doctorate in public health. Her primary interests lie in maternal and child health and the prevention of early childhood caries. She is focused on global health and public health, specifically in relation to children's oral health.

I was introduced to Dr. Cabrera-Matta by our common Alpha friend Dr. Aurora Alva. With the participation of Dr. Cabrera-Matta, the Alphas are extending its coverage to South America, including the particularity and culture of the people of Peru.

"To grow, we must respect one another. Then, and only then, we can learn from each other."
Dr. Bak Nguyen

Well, although Dr. Cabrera-Matta is fluid in English, from the beginning of her interview process, we both concluded that having her to speak in her native tongue would be much more beneficial to our book, as she was asked to answer the questions as if she was in front of patients and their parents.

I don't speak *Espanol*. *Solo un poco*. But thanks to technology, we made it work. So I was listening and accompanying Ailin as she went by the entire list of FAQs we have planned. It was Monday evening and Dr. Ailin started with much energy and enthusiasm. Even if I could only get bits and pieces from her answers, I could feel her passion and how important it was for her to transfer her knowledge and passion to her audience. After close to 2 hours of interview, we were only halfway through.

I suggested a break. She suggested postponing so the 2nd half of her chapter would be of the same quality as the first half. We reconvene for later that week and we went on for another 2 hours! This is how dedicate and committed Dr. Ailin Cabrera-Matta was. That made a huge impression on me.

Dr. Ailin is a Ph.D. in public health on top of being a paediatric dentist. She is super busy, and yet, she took 4 hours out of her busy schedule to help us with the writing of this book, for the benefit of patients all around the world. When I say that I am not giving Alpha titles, only recognizing Alphas and welcoming them into my platform, this is what I meant. Dr. Cabrera-Matta is a true Alpha, one compassionate and engaged in her vocation, dental health and the happiness of her patients.

It is with great honour to introduce to you, Dr. Ailin Cabrera-Matta.

This is **ALPHA DENTISTRY vol. 3, PAEDIATRIC DENTISTRY FAQ**. Welcome to the Alphas.

Dr. BAK NGUYEN

CHAPTER 8
"PAEDIATRIC DENTISTRY"
by Dr. AILIN CABRERA-MATTA
FROM PERU 🇵🇪

8.1 - DEFINITIONS

by Dr. AILIN CABRERA-MATTA FROM PERU 🇵🇪

WHAT IS THE BEST TYPE OF TOOTHBRUSH FOR MY CHILD?

The answer will depend on your child's age and specific needs. For easier understanding, we'll break down the key features of toothbrushes according to children's ages:

Children under six years old:
- Appropriate head size: The toothbrush should have a suitable head size for the child's mouth.
- Two toothbrushes: It's recommended to have one toothbrush for the child and another for the adult who helps them brush.
- Soft and not too long bristles: This makes brushing easier, especially at the back of the mouth and around the molars.

Children over six years old:
- Thick and comfortable handle: The handle should be suitable for the child to grasp properly.
- Soft and not too long bristles: This helps the child brush correctly.

Children with sensitive teeth or enamel defects:
- Extra soft bristles: If your child has very sensitive teeth, such as in cases of molar and incisor

hypomineralization, it's important to use a toothbrush with extra soft bristles.

Additionally, consider the option of an electric toothbrush for children, as it can make brushing easier and ensure proper cleaning. It's also crucial to change the toothbrush regularly, regardless of the type of brush used. Remember that consulting a dentist or expert on the topic can provide additional information and specific recommendations for your child's needs.

WHAT IS THE ROLE OF FLUORIDE IN PREVENTING CAVITIES?
The role of fluoride in the prevention of dental caries is significant, but it is essential to consider other factors that contribute to overall dental health. Fluoride is an important agent in preventing dental caries in both children and adults. However, maintaining proper oral hygiene, adhering to a balanced diet, and having regular dental check-ups also play essential roles in preventing dental caries. Fluoride contributes to dental health in several ways.

First, it promotes the remineralization of tooth enamel, which is the outermost layer of a tooth. Enamel is made up of a complex mineral compound called hydroxyapatite, which can disintegrate under certain circumstances, such as poor dietary habits or environmental factors. This process is known as demineralization. Remineralization, on the other hand, is the opposite reaction, helping to repair and strengthen tooth enamel. Fluoride facilitates remineralization, which can prevent and control existing caries lesions, including early-stage dental caries that may not be visible.

Furthermore, fluoride helps form a stronger protective layer around the tooth enamel by facilitating the formation of crystals or compounds that give strength to the enamel. This "shield" makes it more difficult for demineralization to occur. Fluoride also plays a role in limiting bacterial growth and acid production in the mouth, which can contribute to the development of dental caries. It is crucial to maintain a consistent presence of fluoride in the oral cavity for these benefits to occur. This can be achieved by using fluoride-containing products such as fluoridated toothpaste, fluoride rinses or gels, and professional fluoride applications by dental professionals during check-ups.

While fluoride is generally beneficial for dental health, it is important to consider potential drawbacks and controversies surrounding its use. Excessive fluoride intake can lead to dental fluorosis, a cosmetic condition that affects the appearance of tooth enamel. Moreover, the debate over water fluoridation in some communities highlights concerns about the balance between public health benefits and potential risks.

WHAT IS THE DIFFERENCE BETWEEN A PAEDIATRIC DENTIST AND A GENERAL DENTIST?

Pediatric dentists, like all dentists, begin their education by training as general dentists at university. After completing their dentistry degree, they, along with other dental professionals, can choose a specialty to pursue, similar to how medical doctors specialize in fields like pediatrics, gynecology, radiology, or endocrinology. Dentists can opt for specialties such as periodontics, endodontics, orthodontics, or oral and maxillofacial surgery, among others. To specialize in pediatric dentistry, dentists undergo an additional two to three years of full-time training.

This specialized training equips pediatric dentists with the skills and knowledge needed to address the unique aspects of treating children, including behavior management, development, and creating a positive dental experience for young patients. Courses in pediatric dentistry programs focus on understanding the psychological, mental, social, and physical development of a child, allowing dentists to provide oral health care tailored to each child's growth and development stage. In contrast to general dentists, pediatric dentists are specifically trained to cater to the needs of children, considering not only their oral health but also their overall well-being. However, it is important to recognize that general dentists also possess valuable expertise and skills in dental care for patients of all ages.

Pediatric dentists utilize various tools and strategies to address children's oral health issues, always beginning with the least invasive solutions and escalating to other options when necessary. These strategies may include sedation or general anesthesia to address complex cases or when a child's behavior requires such interventions. Additionally, pediatric dentists have specialized training to manage oral cavity diseases more frequently encountered in children, which may present differently than in adults. They employ strategies to treat common conditions like dental caries using less invasive interventions and requiring less time in the dental office compared to treatments provided by general dentists. By providing specific examples of these strategies, readers can better understand the unique approaches pediatric dentists take to ensure optimal oral health care for children.

WHAT ARE THE MOST COMMON ORTHODONTIC PROBLEMS IN CHILDREN?

The most common orthodontic problems in children involve malocclusions, which are misalignments of the teeth or incorrect bites. Among the various types of malocclusions, class one malocclusion is the most frequent and is characterized by space-related issues. In class one malocclusion, the size of a child's teeth does not match the available space in their upper and lower jaw, leading to problems such as overcrowding or spacing issues. The prevalence of class one malocclusion varies depending on the population, and its causes can be genetic or environmental. For example, if a child has experienced cavities in their primary teeth at a young age, there may not be enough space preserved for the eruption of permanent teeth. Consequently, this results in crowding of permanent teeth, which may require orthodontic treatment to correct.

Another factor that can contribute to orthodontic problems in children is the presence of habits, such as thumb sucking or atypical swallowing. These habits can have long-term consequences for a child's dental health and may lead to malocclusions when their permanent teeth emerge. In addition to malocclusions, children may also experience other orthodontic issues, such as crossbites, overbites, or underbites. It is important for parents and caregivers to be aware of these potential problems and seek professional dental advice to ensure optimal oral health for their children.

HOW CAN I TELL IF MY CHILD NEEDS ORTHODONTIC TREATMENT?

Determining the appropriate timing for orthodontic treatment in children can be complex, as treatments can vary widely. Two main types of treatment include fixed orthodontic treatment with brackets and orthopedic appliances, which can be either removable or fixed. Fixed orthodontic treatment typically involves using brackets to correct misaligned teeth or bites. A suitable time for an initial orthodontic consultation is when the first phase of mixed dentition (a combination of primary and permanent teeth) ends.

This occurs when the first four permanent molars and the eight incisors have erupted, allowing the orthodontist to assess if there is a discrepancy between the size of the teeth and the available space in the child's jaws. Orthopedic appliances, on the other hand, help correct jaw growth and alignment issues. The ideal age for a child's first evaluation for orthopedic appliance treatment is around two and a half to three years old when their primary second molars have erupted. At this stage, a more stable occlusion (the way the upper and lower teeth fit together) is established, and dental professionals can assess if the child's upper and lower jaws align properly.

It is important to note that the American Association of Orthodontists recommends children have their first orthodontic evaluation by the age of seven. This widely accepted guideline ensures that potential issues are identified and treated in a timely manner. While the discussion above outlines two key moments to consider orthodontic treatment, it's crucial for children to have regular dental checkups. These visits provide opportunities for dental professionals to monitor a child's dental development and recommend orthodontic evaluations or treatments as needed. Ultimately, understanding the range of orthodontic treatments available and seeking professional advice will help ensure optimal oral health for children.

WHAT ARE THE BENEFITS OF DENTAL SEALANTS FOR CHILDREN?

The teeth that require dental sealants in children are the molars, specifically the second primary molars in the primary dentition, which are the baby teeth. These molars often have deep grooves and fissures that are difficult for a toothbrush to clean, making it easier for bacteria to accumulate and cause tooth decay. In some cases, it may also be necessary to apply sealants to the first primary molars or even the first permanent molars or premolars, depending on the evaluation of each patient. Applying sealants to these teeth can help prevent tooth decay and the need for restorative treatment, which not only saves money but also makes dental treatment easier for children. With sealants, children only need to come in for preventive maintenance, such as cleanings or reapplication of the sealant, which can improve their acceptance of dental treatment in the future.

8.2 - PREVENTION

by Dr. AILIN CABRERA-MATTA FROM PERU 🇵🇪

HOW CAN I PREPARE MY CHILD FOR THEIR FIRST DENTAL VISIT?

It's important to remember that you should talk to your child's paediatrician before preparing them for any dental procedure. This will help ensure that you have accurate information and don't inadvertently confuse your child. One of the most important things you can do to help your child cooperate during dental visits is to never associate the dentist or the office with anything negative. Avoid using phrases like "if you misbehave, you'll have to go to the dentist" or anything that links dental work with punishment or pain. Instead, have an honest conversation with your child, using language appropriate for their age and developmental level, and explain that dental visits are necessary to help them smile, speak, and eat comfortably. Positive reinforcement, such as promising a fun activity after a procedure, can also be helpful in some cases.

HOW CAN I HELP MY CHILD OVERCOME THEIR FEAR OF THE DENTIST?

Prevention is always ideal when it comes to children and dental care. A child who is afraid of the dentist might have had a previous negative experience, which could have been avoided with a focus on prevention. However, if a negative experience has already occurred or the child has heard about it from a sibling or someone close, there are ways to help them overcome their fear. One approach is to associate dental visits with positive experiences through a process called "sensitization."

During consultations, this involves gradually exposing the child to situations or ideas involving the dentist or paediatric dentist, starting with simple interactions and progressing to more collaborative activities. A child could accompany a parent or sibling who is not afraid of the dentist, visit the dental office as an observer, or be introduced to toys, cartoons, or other materials related to dentistry to become more comfortable with dental procedures.

IS IT OKAY FOR CHILDREN TO CONSUME SUGARY FOODS AND DRINKS?

In an ideal world, children would not consume sugary foods and drinks. However, the key lies in finding a balance and making conscious decisions about their consumption. A child's general and oral health depends on their daily habits and diet. If the family is already focused on a healthy diet that prioritizes fruits and vegetables, occasional treats are acceptable. However, if the child consumes sugary foods and drinks daily, such as in their school lunches, it can lead to the deterioration of their oral and general health. It is crucial to establish guidelines for limiting sugary treats to special occasions or specific times of the day, such as right after a meal, to minimize the negative impact on oral health.

HOW CAN I ENSURE MY CHILD IS GETTING ENOUGH FLUORIDE?

Ensuring a child receives enough fluoride is vital for maintaining healthy teeth and preventing cavities, as fluoride strengthens tooth enamel. There is no specific test to measure fluoride intake, but it's essential to consider the water source in the region. In some countries, like Peru and Latin America, fluoridated water is not available. In such cases, it's crucial to ensure the child gets fluoride from other sources like fluoride toothpaste, mouthwash, or supplements.

Discussing fluoride intake with a dentist or paediatrician is necessary to guarantee the child is receiving enough fluoride. Using toothpaste with the appropriate amount of fluoride is essential for children of all ages, with a minimum of 1,000 parts per million (ppm). The right amount of fluoride in toothpaste ranges between 1,000 and 1,500 ppm. The amount of toothpaste to use depends on the child's age: for children up to three years old or younger than 36 months, use a tiny amount of toothpaste equivalent to a grain of uncooked rice; for children between three and six years old, use an amount roughly the size of a pea. This guideline applies to all children, regardless of whether the water in their country is fluoridated.

If your child is older than six years and has a high risk of cavities, a paediatric dentist can determine this during a consultation by asking questions and examining the child's mouth. Children with a high risk of cavities may need to use a fluoride mouthwash, and the dentist will advise on the amount, frequency, and correct order of application.Remember to use fluoride agents for home use, such as fluoridated toothpaste and mouthwash. Professional fluoride agents, like fluoride gel, foam, or varnish, are commonly used with children today.

The dentist will determine the frequency of these treatments based on your child's risk of cavities. Generally, for low-risk children, treatments will be twice a year, every six months. However, for children with specific circumstances, such as cavities or other conditions that increase their risk, treatments may be required every three or four months, depending on the case.

CAN MY CHILD STILL ENJOY SWEET TREATS WHILE MAINTAINING GOOD ORAL HYGIENE?
Not everything has to be black and white. In dentistry, balance is essential, and it's the daily habits that make the difference. Dental caries is a multifactorial problem, and we strive to tip the balance in favour of your child's dental health by identifying and weighing protective and risk factors during the consultation. If there is

occasional consumption of sweets, it should not be the norm and should be accompanied by proper oral hygiene with an appropriate toothbrush, toothpaste, and the right amount of fluoride. We will also suggest using dental floss and mouthwash as necessary to maintain the balance in favour of your child's dental health.

It is important to analyze all the factors that can impact your child's dental health and be able to recognize them. Some children are born with a higher risk of dental caries due to weakened tooth enamel, mineralization defects, or other reasons. If your child falls into this category, we will suggest increasing protective factors such as appropriate oral hygiene and regular check-ups. In such cases, the consumption of sweets and candies should be more controlled.

HOW CAN I PREVENT ORTHODONTIC PROBLEMS IN MY CHILD?

Malocclusion problems that require orthodontic treatment often have a genetic basis. However, some factors in the environment can potentiate or mitigate them. For instance, if your child has a genetic predisposition for a protruding upper jaw, and they also have a habit of sucking their thumb, the habit will increase the risk of malocclusion. You can prevent this by paying attention to your child's habits, such as thumb-sucking, object-sucking, or pushing their tongue when they swallow. Your paediatric dentist will identify these habits during the consultation and help you prevent them from exacerbating the genetic predisposition.

Another example is when your child has no genetic predisposition for malocclusion, but they have cavities from an early age. This can lead to early tooth loss, and if left untreated, it can cause a lack of space for permanent teeth, requiring orthodontic treatment. Therefore, preventing cavities also helps minimize the risk of orthodontic problems or lack of space for permanent teeth. Primary teeth play an important role in keeping space for permanent teeth in your child's mouth.

Many orthodontic problems have a genetic basis, while others can be influenced by environmental factors. For example, your child may be born with a genetic predisposition for a prominent upper jaw. Additionally, poor habits such as thumb-sucking can further increase the risk of orthodontic problems. We encourage prevention whenever possible, but if your child has a fear of the dentist due to a negative experience, we suggest gradually exposing them to positive experiences associated with dentistry. You can accompany your child to the dentist and allow them to familiarize themselves with the office, equipment, and staff. You can also buy them toys related to dentistry or let them watch cartoons that show positive experiences associated with going to the dentist.

HOW CAN I PREPARE MY CHILD FOR A DENTAL PROCEDURE?
The first thing you need to do is talk to your child's paediatrician and ask them about the procedure and how you can help prepare your child. This is essential because sometimes your interpretation of the procedure may differ from what it actually involves.

HOW CAN I ENSURE MY CHILD IS RECEIVING ADEQUATE NUTRITION FOR HEALTHY TEETH?

First, I must say that nutrition or a healthy diet for healthy teeth is practically the same as what you should do for your child to have a healthy life. So, everything you do to prioritize the consumption of vegetables, fruits, and to have balance in their diet as explained by their pediatrician or nurse, if followed consistently and daily, will help your child have healthy teeth. What I mean is that there is no secret to giving something additional to make their teeth healthier.

Now, if we are talking about their primary teeth, the quality of their primary teeth obviously depends on how the pregnancy and nutrition of the mother was during pregnancy and how the first years of life were, which also plays an important role. I am referring to the first two to three years of life, and what happens in that window of time is important for the child to have good general health and good oral health, including healthy teeth. Therefore, everything that is promoted, including nutrition, care that you give, and the check-ups that you take with their pediatrician or nurse, are vital during their first years of life because the healthier they are, the healthier their teeth will be.

Currently, it is known that children who get sick frequently during their early years of life, for example, with respiratory infections and repeated episodes of fever, may have a higher risk of having some defects in their tooth enamel compared to children who have been healthy. So, everything you do to keep them healthy and have adequate nutrition during the first years of life will be very good for their teeth too.

8.3 - TIME

by Dr. AILIN CABRERA-MATTA FROM PERU 🇵🇪

WHAT IS THE BEST AGE FOR A CHILD TO START SEEING A DENTIST?

Global guidelines and recommendations currently indicate that the first visit to a pediatric dentist should be before the first birthday, ideally in the window of time between when their first tooth erupts and their twelve months of age. During this period of time, it would be ideal to take your child to the pediatric dentist for the first time. Why? Because the idea now is that the child does not have caries, prevention is always the goal, so it is important that we explain everything that you need to do to take care of your child's teeth and mouth so that they stay healthy.

HOW OFTEN SHOULD MY CHILD SEE A DENTIST?

All children should go to the dentist at least twice a year, i.e., every six months. In some specific circumstances, when we identify that there is a high risk of cavities or some other pathology in your child's mouth, we will explain why and recommend seeing them every three to four months. If everything is okay and we are dealing with a child with a low risk of cavities, then taking them every six months at a minimum will be sufficient.

WHAT IS THE BEST AGE FOR A CHILD TO GET ORTHODONTIC TREATMENT?

There is no single answer because each case is different. What is important is that you take your child to a paediatric dentist from an early age, and we will evaluate your child in the office and tell you the appropriate time for evaluation by an orthodontist. In many cases, there are various alternatives. Sometimes, early treatment with removable appliances is necessary, followed by fixed orthodontic treatment with brackets. In other cases, we may wait for more teeth to erupt before initiating orthodontic treatment. Therefore, each case is different, and there is no single age for starting orthodontic treatment.

WHAT ARE THE SIGNS OF TEETH ERUPTION IN A CHILD?

The signs could be constant drooling, increased sensitivity, rubbing the gums with hands, and increased crying. In such cases, it is essential to stay vigilant and consult a paediatric dentist if necessary. If we are talking about a child who is older and starting to have permanent teeth eruption, the signs that first molars are coming in could be complaining of pain at the back of the mouth, avoiding hard foods, and swelling or other visible signs. In such cases, it is necessary to stay attentive and consult a paediatric dentist to determine if it is a normal physiological process or something more concerning.

8.4 - MAINTENANCE

by Dr. AILIN CABRERA-MATTA FROM PERU

WHAT IS THE RIGHT WAY TO CLEAN MY CHILD'S TEETH?
Proper dental hygiene is crucial for maintaining good oral health in children. When it comes to brushing your child's teeth, the approach will vary depending on their age and level of development.

For very young children, aged 36 months or less, it is important to clean their teeth as an adult would. While they may be able to hold a toothbrush and play with it, they likely do not yet have the necessary psychomotor skills to use it effectively. Therefore, it is important for an adult, ideally, the child's parent or caregiver, to brush the child's teeth for them. When it comes to selecting the appropriate toothbrush for your child, there are several factors to consider, such as their age and level of development. However, there are also a few important points to keep in mind when it comes to brushing their teeth.

Firstly, the child should have their head supported during the brushing process. For small children, lying down is often the best position, as it allows for proper support of the head. This can be achieved by laying the child on a bed, sofa, or other surface, or by holding them in your arms. Without proper support, the child may lean back when you try to brush their teeth, making it difficult to clean them effectively. Secondly, lifting the lip is crucial for effective cleaning. A small child may try to use their lips to exert force, which can make it difficult to clean the entire surface of the tooth effectively. Therefore, it is important to lift the upper lip or separate the lower lip to ensure proper access to the teeth.

Finally, the brushing motion is important, as a small child may not have a lot of tolerance. Disrupting the mass of bacteria, called biofilm, that forms on the teeth is essential for maintaining good oral health. Sweeping and circular motions are ideal for disrupting the biofilm and should be used in conjunction with separating the lip. For children between three and six years old, the same three points apply, but the approach can be slightly different. Since they are older, they may not need to be laid down for brushing. Instead, they can stand up, but their head still needs to be properly supported. A mirror can also be used to show the child how to brush their teeth effectively, allowing them to learn and develop good oral hygiene habits.

It is important to follow a specific order when brushing a child's teeth. Starting at the top, move to the outside from right to left, then move to the inside of the teeth. Brushing with sweeping and circular motions is ideal for cleaning each surface of the teeth in the part that's on the palate, which is the back part of the teeth. Keep going until you reach the left side, then move down to the right side again, still on the outside, and keep going from the last tooth, moving forward until you reach the last tooth on the left side. Then go back to the right and brush the part of the tooth that's against the tongue, using the same circular motion. It is important to clean all the surfaces of the tooth, including the parts that are used for chewing. By following these guidelines and brushing your child's teeth effectively, you can help ensure their oral health and set them up for a lifetime of good habits.

HOW CAN I ENCOURAGE MY CHILD TO BRUSH THEIR TEETH REGULARLY?

From a brushing perspective, it's important to note that if your child has teeth that are tightly spaced together, you may need to use floss. This isn't always the case for young children with baby teeth, but many children do require it. If flossing is necessary, the order of the cleaning routine should be flossing first, followed by brushing with toothpaste. If your child is seven years old or older and has been instructed by an odontopaediatrician to use mouthwash, then they should use it as well. This is the general order to follow for proper teeth cleaning.

As for how to encourage your child to regularly brush their teeth, leading by example is the best way. If you brush your teeth every day as part of your routine, your child is more likely to do the same. Additionally, it can be challenging for children to brush for the recommended amount of time, so using timers or small games to help them understand the necessary time commitment can be helpful. Ultimately, it's important to supervise your child's brushing until they are able to do it correctly and for the appropriate amount of time, which will vary from child to child.

To prevent tooth decay in your child's baby teeth, it's crucial to identify any risk factors early on, such as weak enamel. If this is the case, your odontopaediatrician will be able to identify the teeth that require extra attention and advise you on how to monitor them closely. Baby teeth with weak enamel may be more prone to chipping or flaking, leaving areas where bacteria can easily take hold and develop into cavities. Therefore, it's essential to take your child for regular check-ups with an odontopaediatrician as soon as their baby teeth begin to emerge.

HOW CAN I PREVENT TOOTH DECAY IN MY CHILD'S BABY TEETH?

Brushing with fluoride toothpaste, a toothpaste with a minimum of one to one and a half thousand parts per million of fluoride. The amount that your paediatric dentist recommends should be a small scrape on the toothbrush or the equivalent of a small grain of uncooked rice. It's important to brush at least twice a day, especially at night.

The second point is to establish a healthy diet from a young age, minimizing the consumption of sugars, including sugary drinks and foods. Children are not born with a taste for sweets, so the longer you delay introducing sugar into their diet, the better. World guidelines suggest that children should not have added sugar in any of their meals or drinks, at least during the first two years of life. It's difficult to do, but it's an important point and is ideal.

Delaying the introduction of sugar in their drinks and meals as much as possible will help reduce the risk of cavities and other health problems such as obesity and diabetes. It's important to avoid or delay the introduction of sugar into your child's diet.

HOW CAN I PREVENT MY CHILD FROM DEVELOPING DENTAL ANXIETY?

The best way to prevent your child from developing dental anxiety is to avoid invasive procedures. You can do this by establishing good dental habits from a young age at home, so your child only needs to visit the pediatric dentist for easy and preventative procedures such as teeth cleaning, fluoride application, and sealants. Prevention is always simpler, easier for the child to accept, less stressful for the family, and less expensive for everyone. This is the best way to avoid dental anxiety in your child.

Another important point to consider is that research links a mother's or primary caregiver's anxiety during dental visits to the behaviour and cooperation of the child. If you're anxious or nervous about your child's dental care, try to control it so you don't transmit it directly to your child. Don't say or express your anxiety, and be aware of your attitudes and body language. Children can easily pick up on these cues, so it's important to consider this point.

HOW CAN I HELP MY CHILD AVOID DENTAL INJURIES?
Traumatic injuries to primary teeth are common when children start walking and take their first steps. The first years are crucial as this is when most falls or traumas occur, which can involve hitting the lips, teeth, or any part of the mouth. It's challenging to provide specific instructions on what to do or not in these situations, but supervising your child during their early steps and providing a safe environment can minimize the risk of falls or tripping on hard surfaces or stairs while playing or exploring.

Now, let's talk about traumatic injuries to permanent teeth. Children with protruding upper front teeth, the incisors, as explained before, with a slightly more developed upper jaw towards the front, and more prominent central incisors, are more prone to complex traumatic injuries during falls or blows. In such cases, it's important to consult your paediatric dentist for early treatments in coordination with the orthodontist to correct any discrepancies or malocclusions.

HOW CAN I HELP MY CHILD AVOID GUM DISEASE?

When it comes to preventing gum diseases, the determination of whether children need a good brushing and flossing routine will depend on their age and risk level, as assessed by their pediatric dentist. It is important to have a good brushing and flossing routine in areas that require extra attention, as this will help prevent gum diseases. Additionally, using fluoride toothpaste and mouthwash, if needed, can also aid in maintaining good oral hygiene. However, it's important to note that not everyone needs mouthwash, so it's best to consult with a pediatric dentist to determine if it's necessary.

Regular check-ups with the pediatric dentist every six months, or more frequently if needed, are also crucial to detect any gum problems and correct them in time. During these check-ups, the pediatric dentist will assess the child's gum health and provide advice on how to improve their oral hygiene routine, if necessary. With good oral hygiene practices and regular check-ups, children can maintain healthy gums and avoid the discomfort and potential complications associated with gum diseases.

HOW CAN I HELP MY CHILD MAINTAIN GOOD ORAL HYGIENE WHILE WEARING BRACES?

The best way to ensure good oral hygiene during fixed orthodontic treatment, such as wearing braces, is to establish good oral hygiene before starting treatment.

This can be achieved by having regular check-ups with the paediatric dentist who can advise on preventive measures that can be taken at home with the child. It is important to work collaboratively with both the orthodontist and the paediatric dentist during the treatment period, and good coordination between the two doctors is crucial. The child with braces must be periodically evaluated by both dentists to ensure that they receive regular cleanings and fluoride applications.

The child and their family must understand the consequences of not maintaining good oral hygiene during orthodontic treatment, which usually lasts for one and a half to two and a half years or more. They need to understand that biofilm, made up of thousands of bacteria, forms around the braces and between teeth, and produces acids that attack the tooth enamel, making it weaker and more prone to decay and cavities. The child and their family must be taught how to improve their oral hygiene, and sometimes, it's necessary to change the brushing tools during the orthodontic treatment. This process requires patience and must be done regularly throughout the orthodontic treatment.

HOW CAN I HELP MY CHILD AVOID TOOTH SENSITIVITY?

Tooth sensitivity can be caused by various factors, but the most common cause is tooth decay. If decay is not prevented, it can reach deeper parts of the tooth and cause sensitivity. Therefore, preventing decay in the first place is crucial. Regular dental check-ups can provide instructions on preventive measures that can be implemented at home, and the paediatric dentist can recommend preventive measures that should be taken in the office and determine how often they should be done based on the child's case. Enamel hypomineralization is also becoming increasingly common and can lead to increased tooth sensitivity. In some cases, even without cavities, tooth sensitivity can occur, and sealants or restorations may be necessary to cover up areas of lost enamel, sometimes even with crowns or other restorative techniques to prevent the teeth from becoming more sensitive.

8.5 - DENTAL WORK

by Dr. AILIN CABRERA-MATTA FROM PERU 🇵🇪

WHAT ARE THE MOST COMMON DENTAL PROBLEMS IN CHILDREN?

Dental problems are prevalent in children worldwide, and parents must be aware of them to maintain their child's oral health. The most common dental problem in children is dental caries, which ranges from white spots to cavities and can lead to the complete destruction of the tooth. Tooth decay occurs when bacteria in the mouth produce acid that attacks the tooth's enamel, causing it to weaken and break down.

Enamel defects are another common dental problem in children, and hypomineralization of molars and incisors is becoming increasingly common. This condition weakens the tooth enamel, leading to sensitivity and an increased risk of cavities. It can also cause discolouration and roughness of the affected teeth. Malocclusions or misaligned teeth are also common dental problems in children, which can be caused by various factors such as genetics, thumb-sucking, or tongue thrusting. Malocclusions can affect a child's bite, speech, and overall oral health.

Furthermore, three common health problems in children can be related to dental issues. Dental problems can lead to pain, difficulty eating, and even infections that can spread to other parts of the body. Therefore, it is crucial to maintain good oral hygiene habits and visit the dentist regularly to prevent and treat dental problems in children.

WHAT CAN I DO IF MY CHILD HAS A DENTAL EMERGENCY?

The initial step to take when faced with a dental emergency with your child is to seek the assistance of a paediatric dentist as soon as possible. It's usually necessary for an evaluation and radiographs to be taken to determine the extent of the dental emergency. Dental emergencies can often result from traumatic injuries to the teeth, such as falls or blows. If your child has suffered a dental injury but no other injuries to other parts of their body such as their head or nose, and there are no concerns from a medical perspective, then you should take them to see a paediatric dentist immediately. The dentist will assess the situation and take radiographs to determine the extent of the injury, and then prescribe the necessary treatment, which can vary greatly depending on the severity of the injury.

Severe and acute dental pain is another type of dental emergency that requires immediate attention. Though it's becoming less common, it's still important to seek prompt dental care and explain the exact nature of the problem when making an appointment. It's important to differentiate between dental pain and more severe issues that may require immediate medical attention, such as facial swelling, fever, or changes in the child's eating or speaking habits. In some cases, treatment in the dental office may not be enough, and other types of management may be necessary.

IS IT NECESSARY FOR MY CHILD TO HAVE DENTAL X-RAYS TAKEN?

Radiographs are essential in paediatric dentistry to identify dental problems that are not visible during a regular dental exam, such as the roots of teeth and the surrounding bone. Depending on the child's age and dental history, the frequency and type of radiographs may vary. A paediatric dentist will carefully evaluate each child's case and recommend radiographs when necessary while minimizing exposure to radiation through the use of lead aprons and collars.

Radiographs, ultrasounds, and blood tests are important diagnostic tools that allow paediatric dentists and dentists to accurately diagnose and treat dental problems in children. Radiographs, in particular, are necessary to detect dental caries, which can't be seen by visual examination alone. It's important to note that radiographs should only be taken when necessary, and the lowest possible dose of radiation should be used.

The best treatment for dental caries in children depends on the severity of the decay. Early detection and intervention are critical to ensure the most conservative treatment possible. In some cases, a simple dental filling may be sufficient, while more severe cases may require root canal therapy or tooth extraction. Radiographs are essential in determining the extent of the decay and what treatments may be necessary.

WHAT IS THE BEST WAY TO TREAT A CHILD'S CAVITIES?

The best way to treat dental caries in a child depends on the size and depth of the lesion, as well as the child's age. Pediatric dentists have a variety of tools and options available, ranging from minimally invasive procedures like sealants and silver diamine fluoride to larger restorations and crowns made with different materials. There is no one-size-fits-all answer to this question, and your child's dentist will explain the various options and their advantages and disadvantages. Depending on the severity, number, and age of the affected teeth, different interventions, techniques, or materials may be used.

WHAT IS DENTAL SEALANT, AND IS IT NECESSARY FOR MY CHILD?

A dental sealant is a protective procedure used to cover deep grooves and fissures in your child's molars and premolars. These areas can be hard to clean with a toothbrush and can harbor decay-causing bacteria. By applying a sealant material to the tooth's surface, we can create a barrier that prevents decay.

Whether or not your child needs a sealant depends on their individual case and your pediatric dentist's recommendation. We typically recommend sealants for teeth with deep pits and fissures that are difficult to clean with brushing. The decision to place sealants is made on a case-by-case basis, taking into account the extent and severity of tooth decay, among other factors.

Sealants are effective in preventing tooth decay and can help avoid the need for more invasive treatments. While not all healthy teeth require sealants, your pediatric dentist may recommend them if they are necessary.

WHAT ARE THE BENEFITS OF ORTHODONTIC TREATMENT FOR CHILDREN?

Regarding the benefits of orthodontic treatment for your child, there are multiple levels to consider. First, correcting the alignment of their teeth and jaws can improve their ability to chew food and speak clearly. In turn, this can enhance their appearance and boost their self-esteem, potentially reducing the risk of bullying. Proper alignment also facilitates oral hygiene, making it easier for your child to maintain healthy teeth and gums and reducing the risk of cavities. Additionally, orthodontic treatment can prevent future issues like temporomandibular joint disorders, which can be painful and uncomfortable.

IS IT OKAY FOR MY CHILD TO PLAY SPORTS WITH BRACES?

Actually, there's no problem with a child playing sports, especially if they are sports like soccer, basketball, and even swimming. The child just needs to take good care, as with any sport there is always a risk of falling or having an accident. So, they should take the same precautions as a child without braces. In terms of the braces themselves, they won't prevent the child from living a normal life, including participating in sports.

WHAT ARE THE RISKS OF NOT TREATING MY CHILD'S CAVITIES?

The initial stage of cavities in children may not present with any symptoms, such as pain, swelling, or infection, and typically affect the outer layers of the tooth, like the enamel and the first half of the dentin. If left untreated, the cavities will continue to progress and move towards the inner part of the tooth, the second half of the dentin and pulp, causing mild pain when eating certain foods or biting down, which may escalate to spontaneous and frequent pain, especially at night.

If the cavities are still untreated, they can lead to infections ranging from moderate to severe and cause swelling inside the mouth, cheeks, and jaws, and even outside the face. The bacteria causing the infection can spread through the nerve of the tooth into the bone, causing serious health problems, fatigue, fever, and, in extreme cases, can spread to other body parts. Hence, it's crucial to treat cavities in a timely manner to prevent further complications and ensure the child's overall health and well-being.

Apart from the health risks, untreated cavities can lead to difficulties in eating, avoiding certain foods, resulting in poor nutrition and growth, and affect speech and pronunciation, especially if the decay destroys the entire crown of the tooth, creating problems for children still learning to speak and develop language skills. Furthermore, untreated caries can lead to potential bullying, affecting self-esteem and social well-being. Finally, untreated cavities can cause pain and discomfort, leading to missed school days and impacting academic performance negatively. Leaving a child's cavities untreated can lead to various risks that may go unnoticed by parents. It's essential to treat caries lesions promptly to prevent such risks and ensure healthy development for the child.

In their psychosocial development, dental health plays an important role. In general, not treating a child's caries lesions will affect their quality of life and overall well-being. Another aspect to consider is that not treating caries lesions in primary teeth for a prolonged period of time can lead to tooth destruction. This may require more invasive treatments in the dental office, such as tooth extraction. In some cases, if there is severe neglect, the crown of the tooth may break, and the child may not be taken to another paediatric dentist. This can result in a loss of space for the eruption of permanent teeth, leading to malocclusion problems. It is crucial to address caries lesions in a timely manner to prevent such complications and ensure proper development of the child's dentition.

HOW CAN I PREVENT BABY BOTTLE TOOTH DECAY IN MY CHILD?

To prevent tooth decay in a young child, specifically in the first two years of life, which is likely the focus of this question, it's important to note that it's not only caused by the baby bottle, but other factors also play a significant role. However, since this question is specifically about the baby bottle, the first point to mention is that ideally, a child should not use a bottle and should be breastfed with their mother's milk. If this is not possible, then exclusive breastfeeding for six months and then the introduction of solid foods while still breastfeeding is recommended by the World Health Organization. However, if a bottle is used, it should only contain milk without any sweeteners. This means that sugar, honey, and other derivatives should not be added to the milk, as they increase the risk of tooth decay in the child.

Another important point is that the risk of tooth decay in a child is significantly higher when they are given a bottle at night to help them sleep. It's essential to clean the child's teeth before they go to sleep, regardless of whether they have had plain milk, sweetened milk, or any other drink. This means brushing their teeth with a toothbrush and toothpaste, as explained in previous questions, to minimize the risk of tooth decay.

Furthermore, the risk of tooth decay increases significantly when a bottle is used to give milk once the child's molars have erupted, which typically occurs at around 18 months of age. Therefore, it's crucial to pay extra attention to the child's oral hygiene by using an appropriate toothbrush, fluoride toothpaste, and ensuring that there are no milk residues left in the mouth.

To summarize, the best way to prevent baby bottle tooth decay is to avoid the use of a bottle if possible. If a bottle is necessary, it should only contain milk without any sweeteners, and the child's teeth should be brushed before they sleep. As the child's molars begin to erupt, extra care should be taken with their oral hygiene, and they should be taken to an odontopaediatrician for regular check-ups.

HOW CAN I FIND A PAEDIATRIC DENTIST FOR MY CHILD?

This is a great question and the best way to find a paediatric dentist may vary depending on the country. However, I suggest taking your child to a public health establishment for regular check-ups. Health professionals at these establishments can monitor your child's weight, height, vaccinations, and overall health. During the child's early years, check-ups may occur more frequently, especially during the first two years of life. The staff can also provide comprehensive care for your child, including advice on nutrition, growth, and development, and can refer you to other professionals, such as a paediatric dentist, who may be available at the same establishment.

If there are no paediatric dental services available at your health establishment, you can ask your paediatrician, family doctor, or nurse for referrals to dental offices or oral health centres in the area. They can provide a list of convenient options within a reasonable distance. If you are unable to locate a new paediatrician, you can ask for recommendations from family and friends who also have children. They may suggest someone who is conveniently located and provide references. In some countries, a paediatric society may maintain a list of affiliated dentists, which is another way to locate registered paediatric dentists in the area.

Regardless of the option you choose, it is essential to establish a close relationship with the paediatric dentist before your child's first birthday. This is the ideal time between the eruption of the first tooth and the child's first birthday. Within this timeframe of a few months, you should take your child for their first dental check-up and establish a dental home. Similar to a medical home, this is where you will receive care from the paediatric dentist with a frequency determined by them based on the child's needs. They will guide you as a parent and the child towards maintaining good oral health and preventing tooth decay.

HOW CAN I HELP MY CHILD MAINTAIN GOOD ORAL HYGIENE WHILE WEARING APPLIANCES?

This is an excellent question, and the answer is to follow all the instructions given by the orthodontist who fitted the braces. The child's orthodontist or odontopaediatrician may have provided instructions on how to care for the braces, but it's essential for the family to take the child for regular check-ups with the orthodontist, usually every three to six months, to ensure preventive care. During these visits, the orthodontist or other paediatric dentist will check the child's oral hygiene and adapt their cleaning techniques to the braces, whether they are fixed or removable.

Fixed braces require extra attention as bacteria can accumulate more easily, but the orthodontist will explain what kind of brush to use, other additional cleaning tools such as dental floss, special brushes, and fluoride mouthwash, and how to adjust the brushing technique to clean the braces properly. If the braces are removable, the orthodontist will explain how to keep them clean and the maintenance required. They may need to be taken out for cleaning, and the orthodontist will explain how to do this. The first thing parents can do to help their child maintain good oral health during orthodontic treatment is to take them for regular check-ups with the orthodontist, who will provide guidance on oral hygiene and how to clean the braces. The second thing parents can do is to supervise their child closely and ensure they follow the instructions given at home.

8.6 - FEAR/PAIN

by Dr. AILIN CABRERA-MATTA FROM PERU 🇵🇪

IS SEDATION DENTISTRY NECESSARY FOR CHILDREN?

In most cases, no. In very specific cases, yes. Sedation or conscious sedation during dental work is not the first choice for paediatric dentists. We always try to perform dental treatments using non-pharmacological behavioural management techniques, which do not involve giving medications to your child. We will try to establish a relationship with the child, explain what the treatment entails, calm them down, and gradually perform the dental treatment from the simplest to the most complex, without the need for drugs in most cases. This works very well in the vast majority of cases. But sometimes, there are circumstances where dental treatment is necessary.

For the reasons I have explained before, it could be an emergency or trauma, or due to cavities. If we cannot carry out our plan, which is to talk to the child and use a series of behavioural management techniques that are more related to the psychological aspect, we will propose an alternative. The alternative is extreme, which is to go to the operating room with general anesthesia. However, this is not for all cases. There are circumstances where it is possible to avoid going to the operating room with general anesthesia by performing some dental treatments under conscious sedation in the dental office.

Some other paediatric dentists prefer to use deep sedation with the accompaniment of an anesthesiologist in the dental office, not all of them have this approach. However, there are very specific circumstances in which this alternative is proposed to parents. But there are always other options, as I explained before, such as general anesthesia or surgery. So, you can always ask your paediatrician what other alternatives exist.

HOW CAN I HELP MY CHILD COPE WITH TOOTH LOSS?
Losing primary teeth is a normal part of childhood development, as these teeth need to make way for the

permanent teeth that will grow in their place. This usually starts to happen around the age of six, when the permanent teeth begin to emerge and the primary teeth start to move and eventually fall out. It's important for parents to talk to their child about this process, using simple words that the child can understand. Ideally, this conversation should take place before any tooth mobility is noticed.

The lower central incisors are typically the first primary teeth to fall out, and this can happen as early as age five. When you start to notice mobility in your child's primary teeth, it's a good time to talk to them about how their mouth is changing and how their new permanent teeth will be a bit bigger than their primary teeth. This can help your child understand and cope better with the natural process of losing teeth.

In some cases, a tooth may need to be extracted due to dental caries, trauma, or orthodontic treatment. If this is the case, it's important to talk to your child's paediatric dentist to get their opinion on the best way to explain the procedure to your child. Each child is different, and the approach may vary depending on the circumstances. It's important to prepare the child for the extraction, but it's also crucial to use appropriate language and avoid scaring them. Talking to the paediatric dentist beforehand can help you understand the best approach for your child and follow their recommendations. As a parent, you know your child best and can also provide your perspective on what may scare them. The paediatric dentist can provide the appropriate terms and level of detail for the procedure that will take place in the office.

HOW CAN I RELIEVE MY CHILD'S TOOTH ERUPTION PAIN?

This process usually happens around six months old, although it can vary from child to child. While it is generally not very painful, if your child experiences discomfort or pain, it's essential to take them to a paediatric dentist to rule out any issues. If it's a normal eruption process, you can soothe the pain at home by giving your child a cold teething ring specially designed for babies. This will help alleviate the inflammation in the gums before the tooth emerges, making the process more comfortable. However, it's crucial to clean the teething ring properly and ensure it's not too hard, but also not too soft.

In older children, when permanent teeth are erupting, pain is less common, but there may still be inflammation and discomfort. In these cases, it's essential to see a paediatric dentist, who can explain what's happening and provide tips for good oral hygiene, such as using a toothbrush with soft bristles and a small head to clean the inflamed area around the emerging tooth. It's crucial to follow the dentist's advice on brushing techniques, as this can minimize discomfort during the eruption process. In some cases, the dentist may need to perform some procedures to alleviate pain, such as cleaning or washing the area or applying medication. Ultimately, with good oral hygiene and professional advice, you can make the process of tooth eruption as comfortable as possible for your child.

WHAT ARE THE RISKS OF USING TEETHING GELS AND CREAMS?

Paediatric dentists generally do not recommend the use of gels, especially those containing active ingredients or anesthetics, for putting in a child's mouth during the tooth-eruption process, as there are significant risks that could compromise the child's health or life. Although significant risks are not present, applying gels is sometimes not easy to do in a localized way, and using too much gel could cause the child to swallow some of it and become numb in other areas of the mouth. This is not desirable. Therefore, it is not something that paediatric dentists recommend due to the difficult manipulation required. There are natural alternatives on the market, but they do not have much evidence to suggest that they help in any way. In most cases, it is better to let the natural tooth eruption process occur without using gels or creams.

HOW CAN I HELP MY CHILD RECOVER AFTER A DENTAL PROCEDURE?

Well, it depends on the type of procedure that was performed. Most dental procedures are simple, such as cleanings or sealant placements. So, it's important not to convey to your child that the procedure was difficult and that they need to recover from it. Instead, we should reinforce positive behaviour and congratulate them for being a good patient. In cases where more invasive procedures are done, such as surgery or the use of anesthesia, the paediatric dentist will provide specific post-treatment instructions.

Parents need to pay attention to their child after the procedure, especially if anesthesia was used. The effect of the anesthesia will continue after the procedure, and the child may feel numbness or tingling in their cheek, lip, tongue, or other facial areas. They may play with or bite themselves unknowingly, causing injuries that will be felt when the anesthesia wears off. Therefore, it's essential to monitor your child and follow the paediatric dentist's instructions, which may include restrictions on physical activity, exposure to the sun, or heat. The recovery time will vary depending on the type of procedure performed, and following the instructions will help your child have a good post-operative experience.

8.7 - MONEY

by Dr. AILIN CABRERA-MATTA FROM PERU 🇵🇪

WHAT IS THE COST OF PAEDIATRIC DENTAL CARE?

While the cost of dental treatment varies by country and dental office, paediatric dental treatment is generally a specialized service that may cost more than treatment from a regular dentist. However, the benefits of seeking treatment from a paediatric dentist include their specialized training in treating children and providing preventive care, which can ultimately save you money by avoiding expensive dental problems. It's essential to consider all factors when deciding on your child's dental care, including the potential for cost savings in the long run.

Orthodontic treatments may or may not be covered by the state, depending on the country. In Peru, paediatric care is covered to some extent by the public health system, but there is a shortage of dental professionals in these facilities, leading many families to seek private paediatric dental treatment.

ARE THOSE COVERED BY THE GOVERNMENT?

I believe that the answer to this question will be different in each country. I can tell you how it works in the country I live in, which is Peru. Paediatric dental care is covered by the government to a certain extent as a public service, but I must also mention that there are not enough professionals working in these public establishments. So, while it is covered by the government, there are not enough resources to meet the demand.

ARE INSURANCE COVERING CHILD DENTAL CARE?

It varies from country to country. In Peru, public and private insurance covers simple procedures for the treatment of caries and prevention, but more complex procedures such as sedation or general anesthesia are not covered, and orthodontic treatments are rarely covered by private insurance.

8.8 - HABITS

by Dr. AILIN CABRERA-MATTA FROM PERU ❚❚

S THUMB-SUCKING HARMFUL TO MY CHILD'S TEETH?

Thumb-sucking can be harmful to your child's teeth and jaw development, not just their teeth, but also their jaw development, especially if the habit is frequent and intense, meaning they suck their thumb many times a day and with a lot of force. This can cause misalignment of the teeth, particularly the upper incisors, and affect the development of their maxilla (upper jaw). If the habit persists for years, it can loosen the maxilla and affect the way your child bites. It is important to address this habit early on to prevent any potential problems.

If you notice your child sucking their thumb frequently and intensely, it is recommended to seek professional advice from a paediatric dentist or psychologist to establish strategies to minimize and eventually stop the habit. In the dental office, we can explain to your child the effects of thumb-sucking on their teeth and mouth using simple terms that you can reinforce at home. It is not always enough to just talk to your child and encourage them to stop the habit.

HOW CAN I ENCOURAGE MY CHILD TO STOP THUMB-SUCKING?
It is important to monitor your child's thumb-sucking habit, especially if they already have teeth, as it can have harmful effects on their teeth and jaw development. Intense and frequent thumb-sucking can cause misalignment of the teeth and jaw, and may even lead to alterations in their bite. If you observe this habit in your child, it is recommended to bring them to a paediatric dentist who can help establish strategies to minimize or stop this habit, which may even involve seeking the help of a psychologist. It is also important to explain to your child in simple terms the effects of this habit on their dental health during the dental consultation.

HOW CAN I PREVENT MY CHILD FROM GRINDING THEIR TEETH AT NIGHT?
Preventing a child from grinding their teeth at night can be challenging as it may be a normal part of their growth and development. However, if you notice significant wear on their teeth or other concerns, it is

important to bring them to a pediatric dentist for evaluation.

WHAT ARE THE DANGERS OF SHARING UTENSILS AND DRINKS WITH MY CHILD?

Sharing utensils and beverages with your child can increase their risk of cavities if the person sharing has poor oral health, as harmful bacteria can be transmitted through saliva. Therefore, it is recommended to avoid sharing utensils and beverages with your child, especially if you or the person sharing has dental problems.

HOW CAN I HELP MY CHILD AVOID JAW PROBLEMS?

If your child has problems with their teeth and jaw position, it is likely due to hereditary factors. However, there are also some local factors that can play a role. To prevent potential problems, it's important to make sure your child doesn't experience any accidents or blows to the jaw during their early years. Additionally, it's important to pay attention to the timing of your child's tooth replacement and take them to a paediatric dentist regularly to detect and address any dental problems early on, such as teeth misalignment. This can help minimize or even prevent more serious issues down the road.

As for preventing dental problems while your child is sleeping, it's important to establish good oral hygiene habits early on, such as brushing teeth before bed, limiting sugary foods and drinks, and encouraging your child to drink plenty of water. It's also a good idea to make sure your child is sleeping on their back, as this can help prevent tooth decay and other dental issues. If you have concerns about your child's dental health while they are sleeping, it's best to consult with a paediatric dentist for guidance and recommendations specific to your child's needs.

HOW CAN I PREVENT DENTAL PROBLEMS IN MY CHILD WHILE THEY ARE SLEEPING?

The first thing that comes to mind is if the child is a baby and does not have teeth, then I would say to follow the instructions of your pediatrician, as in my opinion, there is no risk from the point of view of their oral health. They can sleep as much as they need to, and as for sleeping positions, you should consult with your pediatrician about which ones to avoid and what is most suitable for your child's case.

Now, if the child already has teeth, it's different. The best thing you can do to prevent dental problems while they're sleeping is to ensure their teeth are clean. When a child is sleeping and there are food residues in their mouth (such as milk), it's the perfect time for harmful bacteria to use that food to produce acids that can attack your child's tooth enamel, whether they have two or four teeth or baby teeth. So, try to get your child into the habit of sleeping with clean teeth. You can give them the appropriate toothbrush and toothpaste and avoid letting them sleep with food or milk residue in their mouth.

This is **ALPHA DENTISTRY vol. 3, PAEDIATRIC DENTISTRY FAQ**. Welcome to the Alphas.

Dr. BAK NGUYEN

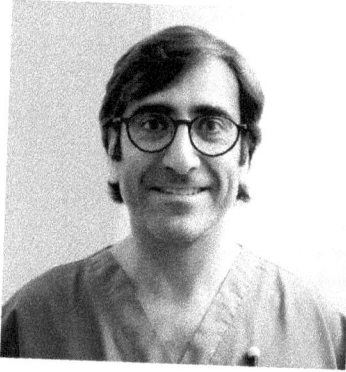

Dr. PIERLUIGI PELAGALLI,
DDS

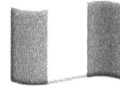

From Italy, ▮▮, **Dr. PIERLUIGI PELAGALLI**, DDS, obtained his degree in Dentistry and Dental Prosthetics from the University of Naples Federico II in 1990. He further specialized in Paediatric Dentistry at the University of L'Aquila and focused his training on periodontology, implantology, and prosthetics. Over the years, he has developed a keen interest in paediatric dentistry and new technologies. Dr. Paelagalli received his periodontal surgery and guided tissue regeneration specialization in 1992 from the Royal Dental School in Aarhus, directed by Professor T. Karring. He attended continuing dental education at New York University and various other specialization courses in Oral Surgery and Fixed Prosthesis. He is a student of Dr. Roberto Olivi for children's dentistry. Dr. Paelagalli has been a professor since 2017 at the Master "Fixed prosthesis on natural teeth and implants" at the University of Rome "La Sapienza." He founded the network "the children's dentist" in 2007, and he is interested in promoting the health of children's mouths. Dr. Pelagalli has published several works, including the classification of implant sites and related therapeutic indications, the advantages of using an Er:YAG laser in pedodontics surgery, Kids Cario Test, and Kids Digital Crown Technique. He is a member of various dental societies and is currently working as a freelancer in Rome.

I met Dr. Pierluigi Pelagalli through the referral of our common friend and Alpha Doctor, Dr. Aurora Alva. I have to express my gratitude to Dr. Alva who has been a tremendous partner, recruiting the best of the best internationally for this team, Alpha 3.

I have to say that it did not take long for Pierluigi and I to connect. Dr. Pelagalli is managing a network of 100 paediatric clinics in Italy. I am so grateful for him to take the time, a Sunday afternoon, to join the Alphas to share his experience and knowledge.

Well, I must say how much fun it was, doing this interview half in English and half in Italian. With international speakers, English is the default language but, getting better at this, and having great A.I. tools at my disposal, I learnt to be more open and flexible. Both of us, appreciate the effort of the other party to make this work. As doctors, as entrepreneurs, as leaders, it reminded us how important it is to stay open and flexible to adapt to any situation. And this is what I learnt from Dr. Pelagalli.

Pierluigi is an experienced dentist who embraced paediatric dentistry later in his career. From there, he built a network of 100 paediatric dental clinics. How many doctors can have such claim? Just like in any of his answers, he is kind, listening, and straight to the point!

I am so grateful to Dr. Pelagalli to have taken the time out of hs busy schedule to share with us. Without further due, please join me to welcoming Dr. Pierluigi Pelagalli.

This is **ALPHA DENTISTRY vol. 3, PAEDIATRIC DENTISTRY FAQ**. Welcome to the Alphas.

CHAPTER 9

"PAEDIATRIC DENTISTRY"

by Dr. PIERLUIGI PELAGALLI

FROM ITALY

9.1 - DEFINITIONS

Dr. PIERLUIGI PELAGALLI FROM ITALY 🔲🔲

WHAT IS THE BEST TYPE OF TOOTHBRUSH FOR MY CHILD?
Choosing the right toothbrush for a child depends on their age. For children under three, it's best to use a very soft and small toothbrush. As the child gets older, toothbrush companies design specific brushes for each age range. Regarding electric toothbrushes, I think they can be a great tool for both children and parents. Electric toothbrushes can make brushing feel like a game, especially for kids who are reluctant to brush. They also ensure a thorough cleaning of the teeth and gums.

WHAT IS THE ROLE OF FLUORIDE IN PREVENTING CAVITIES?
Fluoride is known to strengthen the teeth and is a crucial component in preventive procedures. Instead of the general use of fluoride, topical applications of fluoride are now preferred. This includes fluoride toothpaste and fluoride-containing mouthwashes. It's important that every child uses fluoride to maintain healthy teeth.

WHAT IS THE DIFFERENCE BETWEEN A PAEDIATRIC DENTIST AND A GENERAL DENTIST?
There are several differences when it comes to treating children at the dentist. First and foremost, the approach is different because children are usually unfamiliar with

dental procedures, so it's important to help them feel comfortable and at ease. Prevention is also key, and children need to be taught the importance of coming to the dentist regularly and maintaining good oral hygiene habits. The goal of treatment for children is typically short-term, with a focus on ensuring that their teeth come in and are healthy during their primary years. Special instruments and sedation techniques are often used for children to ensure that they are comfortable during treatment.

WHAT ARE THE MOST COMMON ORTHODONTIC PROBLEMS IN CHILDREN?

The most common dental problems in children are often caused by bad habits such as thumb-sucking, pacifier use, and bottle-feeding. It is important to address these habits early on to prevent future dental issues. Parents and caregivers should be advised on how to help their children break these habits, such as offering positive reinforcement, using a reward system, and gradually reducing the habit over time. Additionally, dentists can provide guidance on appropriate pacifier use and weaning techniques. By addressing these bad habits, we can help children maintain good oral health and prevent future dental problems.

HOW CAN I TELL IF MY CHILD NEEDS ORTHODONTIC TREATMENT?

Orthodontic treatment can help to address both aesthetic and functional problems. As dental professionals, we can explain to parents and children the potential benefits of using orthodontic appliances to achieve a perfect smile and also address functional issues such as bad occlusion.

The importance of identifying if a child needs orthodontic treatment cannot be overstated. Through routine dental checkups, a dentist can evaluate a child's teeth and determine if orthodontic treatment is necessary. We explain to parents the potential consequences of not addressing bad occlusions, such as dental health problems and difficulties with chewing and speaking. It's crucial to motivate children with the potential benefits of treatment, as well as to emphasize the importance of maintaining good oral hygiene throughout orthodontic treatment. Brushing and flossing regularly is crucial to preventing decay and gum disease.

Paediatric dentistry can play a crucial role in identifying orthodontic issues early on in a child's development. By seeing a child from a young age, a dentist can determine if there are any issues with occlusion or the child's smile and face. Although some aspects of treatment can be initiated by a paediatric dentist, the collaboration of an orthodontist is necessary to complete the full scope of orthodontic treatment. As paediatric dentists, we may refer patients to an orthodontist for further evaluation and treatment.

WHAT ARE THE BENEFITS OF DENTAL SEALANTS FOR CHILDREN?
Dental sealants provide many benefits as they can help prevent dental caries. The current trend is to apply sealants to every child, not just those with a high risk of cavities. The way sealants work is by preventing plaque buildup on tooth surfaces, particularly in the deep grooves and fissures of teeth, making them easier to clean. This helps to reduce the risk of tooth decay.

9.2 - PREVENTION

Dr. PIERLUIGI PELAGALLI FROM ITALY

HOW CAN I PREPARE MY CHILD FOR THEIR FIRST DENTAL VISIT?

The first dental visit is an important milestone for children, and parents should approach it positively. Instead of preparing the child with specific details, keep it simple and tell them that they are going to visit a dentist who will check their teeth. Focus on making the experience fun and stress-free. After the visit, reward the child with something special, like a favourite treat or activity. Avoid mentioning any potential discomfort or fear associated with dental procedures to prevent the child from developing negative associations with future visits.

HOW CAN I HELP MY CHILD OVERCOME THEIR FEAR OF THE DENTIST?

It's important to avoid using negative language when talking to children about going to the dentist. Instead, focus on making it a positive experience by using happy and encouraging words. Encourage children to bring their favorite toy or wear their favorite shirt to the appointment, making it feel more like a fun event rather than a scary one.

IS IT OKAY FOR CHILDREN TO CONSUME SUGARY FOODS AND DRINKS?

It is important to follow a controlled diet for children to maintain good dental health. This includes limiting the number of sugary snacks and drinks to a maximum of five times per day. Sugary drinks are a major cause of tooth decay and should be avoided as much as possible.

HOW CAN I ENSURE MY CHILD IS GETTING ENOUGH FLUORIDE?
It's important to choose a toothpaste with an appropriate amount of fluoride for your child's age. In Italy, for example, the recommended amount is up to 1,000-1,450 parts per million of fluoride for children over three years old. If a dentist determines that additional fluoride is necessary, a fluoride mouthwash may be prescribed. As for the risk of overdosing on fluoride, when used properly, the risk is low. However, it's important to supervise your child's tooth brushing and ensure they are not using too much toothpaste or swallowing it. A pea-sized amount of toothpaste is sufficient for children.

CAN MY CHILD STILL ENJOY SWEET TREATS WHILE MAINTAINING GOOD ORAL HYGIENE?
There are two important factors that contribute to good oral health: oral hygiene and a healthy diet. While oral hygiene is crucial, it's equally important to pay attention to what we eat. Consuming excessive amounts of sugary foods and drinks can increase the risk of tooth decay and other oral health issues. Therefore, it's important to maintain control over both factors for optimal oral health.

HOW CAN I PREVENT ORTHODONTIC PROBLEMS IN MY CHILD?
One of the most damaging oral habits is thumb sucking, which is also the most common. It's important to address this habit early on as it can cause misalignment and other orthodontic issues. Other bad oral habits to avoid include tongue thrusting and mouth breathing.

It's important to work on correcting these habits to prevent orthodontic problems from developing in the future. Early orthodontic visits can also help to identify any issues and allow for early intervention to correct them. By taking steps to prevent and correct bad oral habits, we can promote better oral health and prevent more severe orthodontic problems from occurring.

HOW CAN I PREPARE MY CHILD FOR A DENTAL PROCEDURE?

It's important to make the child feel comfortable and at ease during their first dental visit. After the initial visit, there may not be any procedures required. The main goal is to familiarize the child with the dental office environment and help them feel comfortable in the dentist's chair. When any procedures are necessary, they should be approached gradually, starting with the easiest and gradually moving on to more complex procedures. The child's comfort and happiness should always be a top priority during these visits, as this will help them feel more at ease and build trust with the dentist.

HOW CAN I ENSURE MY CHILD IS RECEIVING ADEQUATE NUTRITION FOR HEALTHY TEETH?

Maintaining a balanced and healthy diet is essential for good oral health. While it's important to avoid foods that are harmful to teeth, such as sugary drinks and candy, it's also important to promote the consumption of foods that are beneficial for teeth, such as cheese, milk, and fruits and vegetables. Rather than simply saying no to certain foods, it's important to encourage a balanced and diverse diet that includes a variety of healthy options. This approach ensures that children receive the nutrients they need for good oral and overall health while also minimizing the risk of tooth decay and other oral health problems.

9.3 - TIME

Dr. PIERLUIGI PELAGALLI FROM ITALY 🇮🇹

WHAT IS THE BEST AGE FOR A CHILD TO START SEEING A DENTIST?

It's important to start educating expectant mothers about the dental health of their future children as early as possible. According to guidelines, a child should visit the dentist within six months of the eruption of their first tooth. This visit allows the dentist to recommend preventive measures that parents can take to ensure the child's dental health. Early Childhood Caries is a serious condition where a child experiences tooth decay within the first few months of their life, highlighting the need for early prevention. By starting preventive measures early and scheduling dental appointments for both parents and children as soon as possible, we can promote good dental health from the beginning.

HOW OFTEN SHOULD MY CHILD SEE A DENTIST?

The frequency of dental checkups depends on the child's age and risk of developing oral health problems. Typically, we recommend seeing children for their first dental visit around six months after their first tooth erupts. However, for older children, we assess their risk for dental problems and determine how often they should come in for checkups. Children with a low risk of developing oral health issues may only need to come in twice a year, while children with a higher risk may need to come in for checkups up to six times a year. This individualized approach ensures that each child receives the appropriate level of care based on their unique needs.

WHAT IS THE BEST AGE FOR A CHILD TO GET ORTHODONTIC TREATMENT?

Orthodontic treatment involves several phases. The first phase is focused on the functional aspect and can begin as early as four to five years old, where functional appliances may be used to correct any muscular dysfunction. The second phase is orthopedic, and this can begin around six to eight years old. The final phase involves aligning the teeth and typically begins around 12 years old when all permanent teeth have erupted. These phases are important in ensuring proper alignment and function of the teeth and jaws.

WHAT ARE THE SIGNS OF TEETH ERUPTION IN A CHILD?

Teething is a natural process that occurs as a child's teeth begin to emerge from their gums. The signs of teeth eruption in a child can vary but typically include irritability, excessive drooling, and a desire to chew on objects. The child may also have swollen and tender gums, and some may develop a mild fever or diarrhea. As the teeth continue to emerge, the child may experience discomfort or pain in the gums and jaw, which can be alleviated with gentle pressure or massage. It's important for parents to maintain good oral hygiene during this time by gently wiping the gums with a damp cloth and later brushing the teeth with a soft-bristled brush and fluoride toothpaste. If parents have concerns about their child's teething process, they should consult their paediatric dentist for guidance and advice.

9.4 - MAINTENANCE

Dr. PIERLUIGI PELAGALLI FROM ITALY 🇮🇹

WHAT IS THE RIGHT WAY TO CLEAN MY CHILD'S TEETH?

To help a child with their tooth brushing, one can assist them with the toothbrush or even use plaque-disclosing tablets which reveal areas where plaque remains after brushing. This helps the child learn proper brushing techniques and ensures that they are removing all the plaque from their teeth. Plaque-disclosing tablets are chewable tablets that contain a dye that stains the plaque on teeth, making it visible and easy to remove. By using these tablets, parents can help their children learn proper brushing techniques and improve their overall oral hygiene.

HOW CAN I ENCOURAGE MY CHILD TO BRUSH THEIR TEETH REGULARLY?

Encouraging children to brush their teeth regularly can be a challenge, but there are some strategies that can be helpful. First, make sure your child has a comfortable and enjoyable toothbrush that they like to use. You can also make brushing a fun activity by turning it into a game, using a timer or a toothbrushing app, or brushing together as a family. It's important to establish a routine and make sure that brushing is a part of your child's daily schedule. You can also offer positive

325

reinforcement, such as praise or rewards, for consistent brushing habits. Finally, educate your child on the importance of good oral hygiene and the benefits of keeping their teeth and gums healthy.

HOW CAN I PREVENT TOOTH DECAY IN MY CHILD'S BABY TEETH?

To prevent tooth decay in baby teeth, it is important to establish good oral hygiene habits early on, such as gently cleaning your baby's gums with a clean, damp cloth after feedings and brushing their teeth twice a day with fluoride toothpaste when they emerge. It's also important to avoid giving your child sugary drinks and snacks, and to limit their intake of sticky, starchy foods. Regular dental check-ups and cleanings can also help catch and prevent decay early on. Applying dental sealants and using fluoride treatments can also provide additional protection against decay.

HOW CAN I PREVENT MY CHILD FROM DEVELOPING DENTAL ANXIETY?

To prevent the child from developing dental anxiety, you should familiarize him/her with the dentist and schedule regular check-ups before any problems arise. During these visits, the experience should be made into an event to make it more enjoyable for the child.

HOW CAN I HELP MY CHILD AVOID DENTAL INJURIES?

In order to help a child become familiar with going to the dentist and to prevent injury and tooth decay, it is important to schedule regular check-ups with the dentist even if there are no problems present. Additionally, if the child plays contact sports, it may be necessary to use a mouthguard for protection.

HOW CAN I HELP MY CHILD AVOID GUM DISEASE?

To help your child avoid gum disease, you can encourage them to maintain good oral hygiene by brushing twice a day with fluoride toothpaste, flossing daily, and using an antiseptic mouthwash. You should also encourage them to eat a healthy diet low in sugar and visit the dentist regularly for check-ups and cleanings. If your child is at a higher risk for gum disease, your dentist may recommend additional preventive measures such as fluoride treatments or dental sealants.

HOW CAN I HELP MY CHILD MAINTAIN GOOD ORAL HYGIENE WHILE WEARING BRACES?

To help my child maintain good oral hygiene even with braces, I can teach them how to use a toothbrush correctly and schedule regular visits with the dental hygienist who can assist in cleaning their teeth thoroughly even with the braces on.

HOW CAN I HELP MY CHILD AVOID TOOTH SENSITIVITY?

Tooth sensitivity can be a painful and uncomfortable experience, and it's important to take steps to prevent it. One of the best ways to avoid tooth sensitivity is to avoid consuming foods that can exacerbate it. This includes acidic foods and drinks such as citrus fruits, soda, and sports drinks, as well as foods high in sugar and carbohydrates. Additionally, it's important to maintain good oral hygiene practices, such as brushing and flossing regularly and using a soft-bristled toothbrush. If you do experience tooth sensitivity, it's important to see a dentist as soon as possible to address the issue and prevent further damage. Your dentist may recommend treatments such as fluoride application, desensitizing toothpaste, or even dental restorations to alleviate sensitivity and protect your teeth.

9.5 - DENTAL WORK

Dr. PIERLUIGI PELAGALLI FROM ITALY 🇮🇹

WHAT ARE THE MOST COMMON DENTAL PROBLEMS IN CHILDREN?

The two most frequent dental issues that affect children are cavities and malocclusions. Cavities are caused by the buildup of plaque and bacteria on teeth, which produce acid that erodes the enamel, leading to decay. To prevent cavities, it's essential to maintain good oral hygiene by brushing and flossing regularly and limiting sugary and acidic foods and drinks.

Malocclusions refer to any misalignment of the teeth or jaws that can affect a child's bite and lead to issues with chewing and speaking. If left untreated, malocclusions can also cause problems with the development of permanent teeth. It's important to have regular dental checkups to catch and address any early signs of cavities or malocclusions.

WHAT CAN I DO IF MY CHILD HAS A DENTAL EMERGENCY?

To ensure a prompt treatment in case of a dental emergency, it's crucial to contact my child's dentist right away.

IS IT NECESSARY FOR MY CHILD TO HAVE DENTAL X-RAYS TAKEN?

Dental X-rays may be needed in certain circumstances, such as after an injury or for specific diagnostic evaluations. For children who are over six years old, there may be a need for more detailed assessments.

WHAT IS THE BEST WAY TO TREAT A CHILD'S CAVITIES?

In children, specific materials containing fluoride are used to protect and strengthen teeth from cavities. These materials have a dual action of shielding and fortifying the teeth.

WHAT IS DENTAL SEALANT, AND IS IT NECESSARY FOR MY CHILD?

Dental sealants are a preventive measure that can help in the prevention of dental caries. These sealants are particularly useful in children and can be applied to the biting surfaces of molars and premolars to protect them from decay. By creating a protective barrier on the tooth's surface, sealants can help prevent bacteria and food particles from accumulating in the crevices of the teeth, reducing the risk of cavities. Therefore, dental sealants are a valuable tool in maintaining good oral health and preventing dental problems.

WHAT ARE THE BENEFITS OF ORTHODONTIC TREATMENT FOR CHILDREN?

The benefits of orthodontic treatment are both functional and aesthetic. The functional benefits are the most important as they can prevent further problems after growth. Additionally, the treatment can improve the overall appearance of the teeth, leading to a boost in self-confidence.

IS IT OKAY FOR MY CHILD TO PLAY SPORTS WITH BRACES?
Yes, it is generally okay for a child to play sports with braces, but extra precautions should be taken to protect the mouth and teeth. A mouthguard is recommended to be worn during physical activity to prevent damage to the braces or injury to the mouth. The type of mouthguard used may depend on the type of braces the child has, and it is important to consult with their orthodontist for specific recommendations.

WHAT ARE THE RISKS OF NOT TREATING MY CHILD'S CAVITIES?
Neglecting a cavity can lead to its further progression, ultimately resulting in the destruction of the affected tooth and episodes of pain. It's important to address cavities as soon as they are detected to prevent the need for more invasive and costly treatments in the future. Regular dental checkups can help detect cavities early on and allow for prompt treatment.

HOW CAN I PREVENT BABY BOTTLE TOOTH DECAY IN MY CHILD?
To prevent baby bottle tooth decay, it's important to avoid allowing the child to have prolonged exposure to sugary liquids from a bottle. This can cause the development of cavities in their teeth, leading to tooth decay and potential pain. It's important to avoid giving sugary drinks to babies, including juice or formula mixed with sugar. Additionally, it's recommended to clean the baby's teeth and gums with a clean damp cloth after feeding, and to avoid allowing the baby to sleep with a bottle in their mouth. This can help reduce the risk of tooth decay and promote good oral health in young children.

HOW CAN I FIND A PAEDIATRIC DENTIST FOR MY CHILD?

In Italy, there is a network of paediatric dentists called "Il Dentista dei Bambini." It is easily accessible through their website, which provides a list of all the facilities across the country where parents can find dentists who specialize in treating children's dental needs.

HOW CAN I HELP MY CHILD MAINTAIN GOOD ORAL HYGIENE WHILE WEARING APPLIANCES?

The proper care for braces depends on the type of braces a child has, and it is important to follow the guidance and instructions provided by the orthodontist who manages their treatment plan. The orthodontist will advise on the proper techniques for brushing, flossing, and maintaining good oral hygiene while wearing braces. It is essential for children to adhere to these guidelines to ensure that their braces function properly, and their teeth are protected from decay or damage during the treatment period. Regular appointments with the orthodontist are also necessary to monitor progress and make any necessary adjustments to the braces.

9.6 - FEAR/PAIN

Dr. PIERLUIGI PELAGALLI FROM ITALY ❚❚

IS SEDATION DENTISTRY NECESSARY FOR CHILDREN?

Sedation can be a useful tool during a child's early dental experiences, as it can help make the experience more comfortable and less stressful. Depending on the specific needs and circumstances, different types of sedation may be recommended by the dentist. Sedation can also be beneficial for children with special needs or dental anxiety. However, it is important to discuss the risks and benefits of sedation with the dentist and to ensure that the child's safety and well-being are prioritized. We frequently use conscious sedation during a child's first few dental visits to help them have a more comfortable and positive experience.

It is important to inquire about the potential risks before using any medication or undergoing any dental procedure. Regular preventive measures should be taken to avoid tooth decay. It should also be noted that teeth eruption can be a potential factor in dental health.

HOW CAN I HELP MY CHILD COPE WITH TOOTH LOSS?

You can help your child cope with tooth loss by reassuring them that it's a normal part of growing up and that their teeth will grow back. You can also help them feel more comfortable by providing soft foods and encouraging them to drink plenty of water. Additionally, you can offer distractions like playing games or reading books to take their mind off any discomfort. If necessary, over-the-counter pain relievers can also be used under the guidance of a paediatrician or dentist.

HOW CAN I RELIEVE MY CHILD'S TOOTH ERUPTION PAIN?

There are different ways to help children deal with the pain of erupting teeth. In some cases, specific medications can be used to manage the pain. For younger children, bite devices can be used to alleviate the discomfort of the tooth eruption process.

WHAT ARE THE RISKS OF USING TEETHING GELS AND CREAMS?

Teething gels and creams can have risks such as accidental ingestion, irritation to the gums, and allergic reactions. The use of benzocaine-containing products can also cause a rare but serious condition called methemoglobinemia. It is important to follow the instructions for use and consult with a healthcare professional before using any teething gels or creams on infants or children.

HOW CAN I HELP MY CHILD RECOVER AFTER A DENTAL PROCEDURE?

To help your child recover after a dental procedure, make sure they rest and avoid physical activities for the rest of the day. Give them soft foods and encourage them to drink plenty of fluids. If necessary, provide them with pain relief medication as prescribed by the dentist. Also, keep an eye on them to ensure they don't accidentally bite their lip or tongue while the anesthesia wears off. Finally, follow the postoperative care instructions provided by the dentist to ensure a smooth and speedy recovery.

9.7 - MONEY

Dr. PIERLUIGI PELAGALLI FROM ITALY 🇮🇹

WHAT IS THE COST OF PAEDIATRIC DENTAL CARE?

Although it is true that in general, when it comes to deciduous teeth, there is a perception that the costs of these therapies should be lower for adults. However, in most cases, these treatments are typically considered private healthcare, as the government in Italy provides limited coverage for emergency care and some treatments at government-run facilities. Patients are required to pay a fee for these services. Private dental care for deciduous teeth, on the other hand, is not covered by the government, with the exception of a tax benefit that allows individuals to deduct some of these expenses from their taxes.

ARE THOSE COVERED BY THE GOVERNMENT?

The government in Italy provides limited coverage for emergency care and some treatments at government-run facilities. Patients are required to pay a fee for these services. Private dental care for deciduous teeth, on the other hand, is not covered by the government, with the exception of a tax benefit that allows individuals to deduct some of these expenses from their taxes.

ARE INSURANCE COVERING CHILD DENTAL CARE?

There are very few insurance plans that cover paediatric dental care for children, so most of the expenses are the responsibility of the parents or caregivers.

9.8 - HABITS

Dr. PIERLUIGI PELAGALLI FROM ITALY 🇮🇹

IS THUMB-SUCKING HARMFUL TO MY CHILD'S TEETH?

Thumb sucking can be harmful to a child's teeth and the overall structure of their mouth, especially if the habit persists beyond three years of age. It can cause misalignment of the teeth and affect the development of the jaw and palate. Therefore, it is important to break this habit as early as possible. However, it is not always easy to get children to stop thumb sucking, and it requires patience and encouragement from parents and caregivers. There are various methods that can be used to discourage thumb sucking, such as positive reinforcement, using a bitter-tasting solution on the thumb, or using a thumb guard. It is important to address this habit as soon as possible to prevent potential dental and orthodontic problems later on.

HOW CAN I ENCOURAGE MY CHILD TO STOP THUMB-SUCKING?

Thumb-sucking can cause problems with teeth alignment and the mouth's shape if it continues beyond the age of three. Encouraging children to stop this habit can be difficult, but there are strategies that parents can use. One such strategy is to provide a pacifier instead of thumb-sucking. Parents can gradually reduce the size of the pacifier over time so that the child will eventually lose interest in it. Another approach is to distract the child with other activities, such as playing with toys or reading books. It's important for parents to be patient and persistent in their efforts to help their child stop thumb-sucking.

HOW CAN I PREVENT MY CHILD FROM GRINDING THEIR TEETH AT NIGHT?
It is not possible to prevent children from grinding their teeth at night, as this is an involuntary action often caused by dental occlusion instability. However, this behaviour is generally considered normal and physiological, so there is no need to take action. In most cases, children will stop grinding their teeth spontaneously.

WHAT ARE THE DANGERS OF SHARING UTENSILS AND DRINKS WITH MY CHILD?
Using utensils and sharing drinks with children can lead to bacterial contamination in their mouth. This increases the risk of transferring bacteria from the parent's mouth to the child's mouth. Therefore, it is crucial to recommend to parents the importance of maintaining good oral hygiene and having a healthy mouth. Specific measures can be taken, such as ensuring that parents wash their hands before feeding or giving drinks to children and encouraging them to brush their teeth regularly. Furthermore, parents should be advised to seek dental treatment if they suspect any oral infection or have a history of dental problems.

HOW CAN I HELP MY CHILD AVOID JAW PROBLEMS?
To avoid problems with the jaw, it is important to know that the development of the jawbones is influenced by muscle actions. Therefore, it is necessary to identify and correct any muscle dysfunctions that could cause alterations and problems in the jaw.

HOW CAN I PREVENT DENTAL PROBLEMS IN MY CHILD WHILE THEY ARE SLEEPING?

The issue of a child's sleep hygiene is crucial. It is important for the child to go to bed with clean teeth, without consuming anything containing sugar after brushing at night. However, it is also essential to monitor the child's breathing during sleep, as improper breathing such as mouth breathing could cause dental problems. If the child is found to be sleeping with their mouth open, it is important to investigate the underlying reasons and address them promptly.

This is **ALPHA DENTISTRY vol. 3, PAEDIATRIC DENTISTRY FAQ**. Welcome to the Alphas.

Dr. BAK NGUYEN

Dr. PRRIYA PORWAL,
BDS, MSD

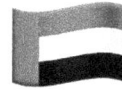

From UNITED ARAB EMIRATES , **Dr. PRRIYA PORWAL,** BDS, MSD, is a paediatric dentist practicing in Abu Dhabi since 2019. She has developed an interest in psychology and clinical hypnotherapy, which she applies to help manage anxiety and uncooperative behaviour of her patients. She has been awarded the Indian Health Professional Awards 2020 for Excellence in Pedodontics. She has been privileged to work with the team of Oncology department in Burjeel Medical City, Abu Dhabi, UAE; as a Specialist Pediatric Dentist, doing Full Mouth Rehabilitation for children requiring Bone Marrow Transplant. . Additionally, she has a strong passion for art, which plays a significant role in her life and influences her approach to dentistry.

Dr. Porwal and I met online. She reached out by liking one of my latest recognitions, my coverage by Brainz Magazine. I have to say how flattered I was to have likes from strangers on LinkedIn. Then, I remembered that this was how I started my rise, reading out to strangers on LinkedIn during the Pandemic. I did not sit long on the satisfaction and reached back.

Well, Prriya was really surprised that I reached back. She did not expected that. As we connected, I discovered a young practionneer full of energy and of hope for the future of our kind. I usually invited experience more than youth to join the Alphas, but meeting with Prriya reminded me important it is to balance both: wisdom and hope.

Compassionate and passionate, Dr. Porwal stands for the future of our profession. After our defeat in covid, being benched and the hard realization of how the rest of the world sees dentistry, I have hope, connecting with the next generation of dental professionals led by doctors like Dr. Porwal.

Without further due, please join me to welcoming Dr. Prriya Portal from the United Arab Emirates.

This is **ALPHA DENTISTRY vol. 3, PAEDIATRIC DENTISTRY FAQ**.
Welcome to the Alphas.

Dr. BAK NGUYEN

CHAPTER 10

"PAEDIATRIC DENTISTRY"

by Dr. PRRIYA PORWAL

FROM UNITED ARAB EMIRATES

10.1 - DEFINITIONS

by Dr. PRRIYA PORWAL FROM UNITED ARAB EMIRATES

WHAT IS THE BEST TYPE OF TOOTHBRUSH FOR MY CHILD?

Using a toothbrush with a small head and soft bristles is recommended. The small head allows you to reach the posterior part of your child's mouth and effectively clean the distal surfaces of the teeth. Choosing a toothbrush with the smallest head is something I would recommend, even for adults. It can be particularly helpful when there is limited mouth opening, allowing you to reach the most difficult areas.

An electric toothbrush can be seen as something new and interesting. If a child is not fond of brushing, using an electric toothbrush can help motivate them. It can also be beneficial for children who may have limited dexterity. However, it's important to note that you can't solely rely on an electric toothbrush. You still need to cover all the surfaces of the teeth and ensure that the toothbrush is properly angled and used correctly. It's not enough to simply place it in one spot and expect it to do all the work. So yes, supervision is required when using an electric toothbrush too. You can introduce it as something fun and novelty for the child, using the electric toothbrush as part of their dental care routine in the morning and evening.

WHAT IS THE ROLE OF FLUORIDE IN PREVENTING CAVITIES?

Firstly, it's one of the simplest procedures and can be done regularly. Fluoride works by altering the structure of the tooth during its development and formation stage and making the tooth enamel stronger. It forms a compound called fluorapatite, which is more resistant to acid attacks. This helps in preventing cavities, even in the early stages when the surface of the tooth is still intact. Fluoride can even halt the progression of early cavities. So, it plays a crucial role in cavity prevention.

WHAT IS THE DIFFERENCE BETWEEN A PAEDIATRIC DENTIST AND A GENERAL DENTIST?

As per the educational aspect, Pediatric Dentists invest additional three years for specializing in the subject, where in they are trained to deal with children with special health care needs, too. They specialize in oral healthcare, from the age of zero to 18 years. As per treatment approach, unlike general dentists who may opt for tooth extraction as a common approach, paediatric dentists take a more comprehensive view. They consider the long-term effects and potential consequences of treatment options. For instance, after tooth extraction, a paediatric dentist recognizes the importance of space maintenance and ensures it is not overlooked.

This is crucial in preventing future issues like space loss and orthodontic problems. Paediatric dentists understand the significance of primary teeth and make every effort to preserve them. Their immediate goal is to retain the tooth and maintain space in the mouth whenever possible. Extraction is always the last resort and is only considered when the prognosis is uncertain.

deep fissures smoother, creating a self-cleansing area. This provides relief during brushing and rinsing, knowing that nothing is getting trapped in those hard-to-reach areas. The accumulation of debris in these fissures is a common starting point for cavities in the first permanent molars, which are particularly vulnerable as they are still undergoing mineralization after the eruption. By sealing these fissures, we ensure that the bacteria have fewer hiding spots and reduce the risk of cavities in these vulnerable areas.

Sealants can sometimes become fractured. It is important to have regular follow-up visits with your dentist, especially a paediatric dentist, every 6 months. During these visits, the dentist will check the condition of the sealants. Factors such as eating habits and diet can influence the longevity of sealants. If they are no longer in place, they can be easily replaced. Redoing the sealants when necessary is the best approach to maintain their effectiveness.

10.2 - PREVENTION

by Dr. PRRIYA PORWAL FROM UNITED ARAB EMIRATES

HOW CAN I PREPARE MY CHILD FOR THEIR FIRST DENTAL VISIT?

Nowadays, there are many YouTube videos featuring dental clinics or dental visits. You can allow your child to watch these videos to familiarize them with the concept. Additionally, having a toy dental kit at home can provide a playful way to introduce dental tools and procedures to your child. By engaging in these activities, you can create a positive and enjoyable experience for your child. If your dentist has an online presence, like my Instagram account, I encourage parents to show their children the pictures and videos on the account. Seeing other children smiling, happy, and enjoying their dental visits can help alleviate anxiety. By becoming familiar with the dentist's face through the online content, the child will feel more comfortable during their actual visit.

To further motivate them, I have created a highlight on my Instagram called "Star Kids." I inform parents that if their child is brave during the dental visit, I will feature their picture in that highlight so that other kids can see how courageous they are. Please note that these suggestions are what I advise to the parents of my patients who may have concerns or anxieties about dental visits.

HOW CAN I HELP MY CHILD OVERCOME THEIR FEAR OF THE DENTIST?

It is important to refrain from sharing any negative dental experiences in front of your child, even if you had a bad experience in the past. Just because you may have had a negative experience does not mean your child will have the same. Avoid discussing negative dental experiences with others when your child is present, as they might overhear and internalize those fears. Even if they seem engaged in another activity, children are sensitive to their surroundings and can pick up on your conversations.

Furthermore, it is crucial not to use scare tactics or threats related to dentists or doctors. Avoid statements like, "If you misbehave, the dentist will give you a shot."

Such statements can create unnecessary anxiety and make dental visits more challenging for both the child and the dentist. Instead, focus on positive and encouraging messages. Promote the importance of dental care and highlight the role of dentists in keeping their teeth healthy, without using fear-based approaches.

If you had a negative dental experience, it is best to create a positive narrative for your child. You can share a made-up story about how a dental visit helped you or emphasize the importance of taking care of your teeth. By promoting positive dental experiences and avoiding negative associations, you can help your child develop a healthy and confident attitude toward dental care. Remember, paediatric dentists are here to care for and support your child, not to remove their teeth.

IS IT OKAY FOR CHILDREN TO CONSUME SUGARY FOODS AND DRINKS?
It is important to limit the consumption of sugary foods and drinks for your child's dental health. Rather than completely depriving them of sweets, opt for sugar-free alternatives available in the market. When it comes to chocolates, it is preferable to choose dark chocolate over milk chocolate as it creates a less acidic environment in the mouth. Dark chocolate is not only considered healthier overall but also better for dental reasons.

To manage the frequency of sugary intake, it is advised to increase the time intervals between consumption. Rather than giving one chocolate every hour, allow your child to have all the chocolates together and then encourage rinsing or brushing afterwards. This approach allows the acid level in the mouth to decrease more effectively. After consuming sugary treats, it is beneficial to provide your child with fruits, vegetables, or cheese to help clean their teeth. Sticky foods like jelly or chewy chocolates should be avoided as they tend to stick to the teeth, making them difficult to remove even with brushing.

Introducing sugar-free options to your child from a young age can help them develop a preference for these alternatives. By gradually reducing their exposure to sugary tastes and promoting sugar-free gum or sweets, they can appreciate the taste of these alternatives without craving excessive amounts of sugar. In terms of drinks, it is best to choose natural options and avoid colas and sodas, which are not suitable for children's consumption. Encouraging the intake of water, milk, or unsweetened beverages is a healthier choice for their overall well-being and dental health.

HOW CAN I ENSURE MY CHILD IS GETTING ENOUGH FLUORIDE?

One aspect to consider is the fluoride content in your water supply, which can vary by region. You can research or inquire about the fluoride levels in your local water and discuss it with your dentist to determine if the amount is appropriate for your child's dental health. Excessive fluoride can have negative effects on teeth, so it is essential to ensure the levels are within the recommended range. If your water supply does not contain fluoride or if you want to supplement your child's fluoride intake further, you can also examine the ingredients of the products they consume. This includes checking the labels of drinks, energy drinks, or other beverages to see if they contain fluoride. By being aware of the fluoride content in these products, you can make informed decisions about your child's fluoride intake.

It is advisable to have a discussion with your dentist to assess your child's specific needs and determine if additional fluoride sources such as fluoride toothpaste or mouthwash are necessary. Your dentist can provide personalized recommendations based on your child's oral health and fluoride requirements. While water is commonly the main source of fluoride, it is crucial to evaluate the specific circumstances and consult with a dental professional for tailored guidance.

CAN MY CHILD STILL ENJOY SWEET TREATS WHILE MAINTAINING GOOD ORAL HYGIENE?

Sugar-free sweets can be a challenge to deal with, as children often have a strong desire for sugary treats. It's common to encounter questions about how to manage this situation. One suggestion is to stock your kitchen cabinets with sugar-free sweets. This way, even if they indulge in a sweet treat, it will be a healthier option without the harmful effects of sugar. Additionally, there are various biscuits, chocolates, and traditional sweets available specifically designed for individuals with diabetes or those seeking sugar-free alternatives.

When you're on the go and your child craves sweets, it's helpful to have some on-the-go, dental cleaning and protecting products readily available. Consider providing vegetables like carrots or fruits like apples, as they can be satisfying and provide a fibrous option, which would help teeth get rid of the sticky sweets. Cheese is also an excellent choice, as it helps regulate the acidic levels in the mouth and mitigates the negative effects of sugary and acidic treats, which can contribute to tooth decay. Encouraging your child to chew on cheese or consume fibrous fruits and vegetables after consuming sweets can help counteract the potential damage caused by the acid and plaque buildup.

It's important to establish a habit of rinsing the mouth after consuming carbohydrates or any food in general. This practice can help maintain oral hygiene and minimize the risk of cavities. By breaking the chain of acid buildup, plaque formation, or bacterial growth, we can effectively prevent cavities from developing. To summarize, incorporating sugar-free alternatives, such as stocking the kitchen with appropriate sweets, offering fibrous fruits and vegetables, and promoting rinsing after eating, can contribute to better oral health and reduce the negative impact of sugary treats on your child's teeth.

One additional suggestion I would like to add, is the option of sugar-free chewing gums. These can be given to children who are older, around seven or eight years old, and who can perform the maneuver of chewing and spitting out a chewing-gum. Sugar-free chewing gums, particularly those containing xylitol, are beneficial for maintaining good oral hygiene. They are a cool and enjoyable way for kids to keep their mouths busy while promoting saliva production, which helps cleanse the teeth and neutralize acids. It's important to ensure that the chewing gum is sugar-free and contains xylitol for optimal dental benefits. By incorporating sugar-free chewing gums into your child's routine, you can offer them an additional tool for maintaining oral health. However, it's essential to supervise younger children to ensure they don't swallow the gum and that they understand proper gum-chewing etiquette.

HOW CAN I PREVENT ORTHODONTIC PROBLEMS IN MY CHILD?

Regular visits to your paediatric dentist are essential in preventing oral health issues. Your paediatric dentist can anticipate potential problems and guide you on taking appropriate steps in a timely manner. The first dental visit should ideally occur around your child's first birthday or when their first tooth erupts. From then on, your paediatric dentist will keep you informed about when to schedule the next visit and what to expect.

During these visits, your dentist will provide you with valuable tips and guidance. They will educate you on important matters such as weaning off bottles and addressing orthodontic concerns that may arise. It is crucial not to prolong bottle use beyond the appropriate age or rely on pacifiers excessively. Your dentist will inform you about the proper timing for discontinuing these habits. To stay well-informed, it is necessary to either educate yourself thoroughly or regularly consult your dentist, who will provide you with age-specific information and guidance.

HOW CAN I PREPARE MY CHILD FOR A DENTAL PROCEDURE?

Regular visits to your paediatric dentist are crucial for maintaining good oral health. Your dentist can anticipate potential issues and guide you on taking the necessary steps at the right time. It is recommended to schedule the first dental visit around your child's first birthday or when their first tooth emerges. From there, your dentist will keep you informed about follow-up appointments and provide valuable insights. During these visits, your dentist will offer helpful tips and advice. They will educate you on important topics such as weaning off bottles and addressing orthodontic concerns. It is important to discontinue bottle use and pacifiers appropriately to prevent oral health issues. Your dentist will provide guidance on the ideal timing for these transitions. Staying informed either through self-education or regular consultations with your dentist is essential.

When preparing your child for dental procedures, it is beneficial to make it a fun and engaging experience. Explain the procedure in a child-friendly manner, such as mentioning the use of a tiny mirror to examine their teeth. Let them know about the water-spraying nozzle and the "Mister Thirsty" straw that helps remove water from their mouth. When discussing fillings, use creative analogies to make it relatable and exciting. For instance, you can create a playful scenario where you and your child are a team fighting against bacteria, with the dental drill as a "machine gun." Emphasize their role in keeping their mouth open while you take care of the rest.

If a local anesthesia shot is involved, use gentle language to describe the sensation. Explain that it will feel possibly warm or ticklish, and compare it to a unique balloon sensation on their cheek. Reassure them that this balloon is special and will disappear on its own after a couple of hours. Encourage them to be careful not to bite or burst the "balloon." By using positive and creative language, you can alleviate your child's concerns and make their dental experience more enjoyable.

In addition, it is essential to prepare your child for a dental procedure involving nitrous gas, commonly known as laughing gas. You can explain to your child that they will experience a sweet flavour, but it will be different as it will be inhaled through their nose rather than consumed orally. Create excitement within your child, by informing them that they with be given the option to choose their preferred flavour. Sharing these insights with you allows you to understand the techniques used to make dental visits more enjoyable for children.

HOW CAN I ENSURE MY CHILD IS RECEIVING ADEQUATE NUTRITION FOR HEALTHY TEETH?

Discussing your child's diet with the dentist is important to address any misconceptions and ensure they are receiving adequate nutrition for healthy teeth. It is crucial to provide detailed information about your child's diet so that the dentist can assess whether they are consuming foods that promote dental health. This discussion will help dispel myths and provide accurate guidance.

10.3 - TIME

by Dr. PRRIYA PORWAL FROM UNITED ARAB EMIRATES

WHAT IS THE BEST AGE FOR A CHILD TO START SEEING A DENTIST?

To maintain good oral health, it is recommended to take your child to the dentist as soon as their first tooth appears. This typically happens during the first year of their life, preferably around their first birthday. By introducing them to the dentist early on, it becomes a regular and familiar experience for the child, alleviating any fear or anxiety associated with dental visits. It is crucial to choose a qualified paediatric dentist who understands the significance of the first dental visit. The initial encounter leaves a lasting impression on the child, influencing their perception and future willingness to seek dental care. Therefore, it is the responsibility of the paediatric dentist to ensure that the first visit is a positive and pleasant experience for the child, as it shapes their attitude towards dental appointments in the future.

HOW OFTEN SHOULD MY CHILD SEE A DENTIST?

It is important to visit the dentist every 6 months for various reasons. Regular check-ups ensure that existing fillings are intact and in good condition, reducing the likelihood of requiring new fillings. Additionally, during these visits, fluoride treatment is provided to maintain optimal oral health. Moreover, thorough monitoring of teeth movements allows for early detection of potential orthodontic issues, helping to determine whether future orthodontic treatment may be necessary. By adhering to a 6 month dental visit schedule, you can stay proactive in maintaining your oral well-being.

WHAT IS THE BEST AGE FOR A CHILD TO GET ORTHODONTIC TREATMENT?

Around the age of 8 to 9, children experience a stage called mixed dentition, during which their primary teeth coexist with the eruption of permanent teeth. This period marks a crucial and dynamic phase of jaw development. It is important to differentiate between interceptive or preventive orthodontics, such as space maintainers or retainers, and braces. The need for such interventions depends on various factors, such as the specific dental issue, the age of tooth extraction, and the anticipated time for the eruption of new teeth.

Space maintainers are utilized when there is a significant time gap between tooth extraction and the emergence of a permanent tooth. Conversely, space regainers may be required if a space maintainer was not initially used, leading to space loss or in case of space-loss due to any other reason. The decision regarding the appropriate age and treatment stage is made by the dentist or paediatric dentist, considering factors like the number and location of teeth being extracted. There are some more appliances whichh are commonly used, like, Hawley's plate, palatal expanders, 2 x4 , etc, depending on the requirement. Some of these can have an option of being removable or fixed.

In the case of braces, it is advisable to consult an orthodontist around eight years of age to assess the child's dental condition and determine the most suitable course of action. Depending on the orthodontist's recommendation, treatment may commence during the mixed dentition phase when both primary and permanent teeth are present or after the primary teeth have naturally fallen out and only permanent teeth remain. Therefore, visiting an orthodontist between the ages of 7 to 9 is typically recommended.

WHAT ARE THE SIGNS OF TEETH ERUPTION IN A CHILD?

Teething symptoms can vary among children, particularly when their primary teeth are erupting. Each child may experience different signs, with some displaying more pronounced symptoms such as fever and diarrhea. Excessive drooling is a common indicator, especially in infants and toddlers who have limited means to express their discomfort. Persistent crying and a tendency to put their fingers in their mouth are additional signs that they are aware of the teething process and the irritation it may cause. While drooling is the most commonly observed symptom, a few children may also develop mild rashes. It is crucial for parents to recognize these symptoms and provide appropriate care and comfort to ease any discomfort associated with teething.

Furthermore, parents may occasionally notice a blue-coloured bulge on their child's gum, referred to as a tooth erupting hematoma, as their new teeth emerge. Although this bulge may initially raise concerns, it is typically not a cause for serious worry. Instead, it can be seen as an indication that the new tooth is growing in a natural and healthy way. It is important to exercise patience while waiting for the tooth to fully erupt. If you have any concerns or doubts, it is advisable to seek confirmation from your dentist, as they are the most qualified professionals to provide accurate information and guidance. It is worth noting that the presence of a blue bulge on the gum is an occasional occurrence and is generally considered a normal part of the teething process.

by Dr. PRRIYA PORWAL FROM UNITED ARAB EMIRATES 📧

WHAT IS THE RIGHT WAY TO CLEAN MY CHILD'S TEETH?

When brushing, use circular motions with the bristles, focusing on vertical rather than horizontal scrubbing. This ensures the effective removal of food particles and thorough cleaning of all tooth surfaces. Even before teeth erupt, clean the gums and tongue using gauze wrapped around your finger. After teeth emerge, switch to a silicone or soft bristle finger brush, paying attention to all areas, including the gums, tongue, and back molars. Begin with a finger brush for control and comfort. Brush for 2 minutes. Use mild-flavoured toothpaste in appropriate amounts: smear-sized for under 3 years old, and rice grain-sized for 3 to 6 years old. Low-concentration fluoride toothpaste is safe. After brushing, spit out excess toothpaste without rinsing to allow it to work effectively.

HOW CAN I ENCOURAGE MY CHILD TO BRUSH THEIR TEETH REGULARLY?

Make brushing a habit by involving your child. Let them watch while you brush your own teeth. Hand them their own toothbrush and let them give it a try. Maintain a positive attitude and make it fun. You can use sand timers or play two-minute videos with their favourite cartoons on YouTube that guide them through brushing each quadrant. These videos often include songs and even promote flossing. Lead by example and let them observe as actions have a greater impact on children than words. Encourage role-playing by demonstrating the habits you want them to develop. Additionally, consider incorporating novelty into their dental routine. Get them toothbrushes in different colours, their favourite cartoon characters, or unique shapes. Electric toothbrushes can also be appealing. Allowing them to choose their toothbrush fosters a sense of ownership and enthusiasm.

HOW CAN I PREVENT TOOTH DECAY IN MY CHILD'S BABY TEETH?

To maintain good dental health, consider important aspects like diet, oral hygiene, and preventive care. Limit consumption of refined and sugary foods, opting for raw and healthier alternatives. Ensure teeth have sufficient space for effective cleaning, including flossing. Cavities often develop between teeth when there isn't enough space for self-cleansing. Flossing is essential, even during primary dentition, and parents should assist if needed. Cavities may go unnoticed as visible tooth surfaces appear clean, but decay can be happening between teeth, requiring X-rays or causing sudden pain.

Regular flossing helps prevent advanced cavities. If teeth surface touch or overlap, flossing is crucial. Practice regular tongue cleaning, brushing, and use appropriate toothpaste and mouthwash. Mild bubble gum or fruit-flavoured products are suitable for children who dislike minty flavours. Tooth Mousse is effective when used nightly to prevent decay and is beneficial for all children. In-office preventive treatments include cleanings, fluoride treatments, and professional care performed by a dentist. Regular dental visits every 6 months are significant for the early detection and intervention of cavities. Unfortunately, cavities cannot heal naturally as enamel lacks self-healing abilities. To restore tooth health and function, cavities must be filled by a dentist. But If the decay Is at Its Initial stage, and cavitation has not happened yet, It could be controlled from becoming a cavity by regular In-office care like topical Fluoride treatment and judicious home dental care.

HOW CAN I PREVENT MY CHILD FROM DEVELOPING DENTAL ANXIETY?

Make dental visits as a normal 3 monthly routine since the age of 1 year or lesser. Aim to visit a Pediatric Dentist particularly, as they know the significance of a first dental visit. Hence, they make sure, It Is a pleasant experience for a kid. In fact, a Pediatric Dentist would make the best of any visits even If that includes a normal check-up, as we certainly want to imbibe a good impression on kids and want them to see us again with a positive attitude. Suddenly, or when In pain, taking a kid to a dentist could fill the mind and heart of the kid with multiple scenarios, possibilities. Whereas, If It Is a routine, they would look forward to It with no botheration. Also, speak to your paediatric dentist before the appointment for any preparation that you could do before taking your kid to the clinic.

HOW CAN I HELP MY CHILD AVOID DENTAL INJURIES?

The sport your child participates in is crucial to consider. Mouth guards are highly recommended, which your dentist can custom-make for your child. They separate the upper and lower teeth arches while providing cushioning in between. Mouth guards also protect the tongue and prevent collisions that could result in fractures. If your child is involved in sports or outdoor activities, using a mouth guard is essential. It's important to note that dental injuries are often observed when children start walking, typically between the ages of two to four. During this time, accidents may occur as they fall, such as hitting tables or other objects. Although it's challenging to prevent such incidents, being attentive is necessary. Additionally, if your child's front teeth, particularly the upper incisors, protrude, they are more susceptible to fractures due to their prominence. In such cases, it is advisable to consult your dentist and take the necessary precautions. These measures significantly contribute to preventing dental injuries in your child.

HOW CAN I HELP MY CHILD AVOID GUM DISEASE?

It's important to maintain oral hygiene for your child. Additionally, consider incorporating gum massage into their regular oral care routine. Massaging the gums stimulates the release of crevicular fluid, which cleanses the area between the gum and the tooth, reducing bacterial accumulation. Regular professional cleanings are also beneficial. Some children have higher mineral content in their saliva, leading to tartar buildup, particularly on the inner side of the lower front teeth. Over time, this can create gaps between the gum and the tooth surface.

Regular flossing and thorough brushing can help prevent the build-up of tartar. If your child has excessive mineral levels in their saliva, regular professional cleanings are necessary, in addition to proper brushing. While accurate and effective brushing can minimize deposits, it's advisable to err on the side of caution. Visit your dentist for regular professional cleanings and ensure regular gum massages at home. Additionally, incorporating vitamin C into their diet can support overall oral health.

HOW CAN I HELP MY CHILD MAINTAIN GOOD ORAL HYGIENE WHILE WEARING BRACES?

Maintaining oral hygiene becomes more challenging with braces. It's important to use a toothbrush with the smallest head size. Since traditional flossing may not be possible, orthodontic toothpicks or interdental brushes can be used to clean food particles stuck between the brackets, wire, and teeth. This may take a bit more time, but it should become a habit. One can use a water-flosser too to do a quick cleaning. Regular brushing with a small head toothbrush and using interdental cleaning aids is essential.

Additionally, if your child is undergoing braces treatment, consider having fluoride treatments every three months instead of every six months. This frequency helps protect against an increased risk of cavities. Topical fluoride varnish treatments can be beneficial. It's important to consult with your dentist regarding the specific recommendations for your area, but as a general guideline, a three-month interval is advisable. Regular professional cleanings are also recommended.

HOW CAN I HELP MY CHILD AVOID TOOTH SENSITIVITY?

Tooth sensitivity can occur due to various reasons. It may be natural if the enamel layer is thin, which is often a genetic trait. In such cases, using desensitizing toothpaste regularly can help manage sensitivity, although consistent use is necessary. If the sensitivity is severe, options like crowns or caps can be considered. However, it is usually preferable to pursue minimally invasive treatments and reserve such interventions for when the child is older. Another common cause of sensitivity is tooth decay. If a cavity is present, it can lead to sensitivity, especially to certain foods. Addressing the cavity through timely dental fillings is crucial as it prevents the exposure of dentin, which can make the tooth extremely sensitive to cold temperatures. In summary, tooth sensitivity can be managed through desensitizing toothpaste, dental interventions like crowns or caps, and addressing any underlying tooth decay promptly.

10.5 - DENTAL WORK

by Dr. PRRIYA PORWAL FROM UNITED ARAB EMIRATES

WHAT ARE THE MOST COMMON DENTAL PROBLEMS IN CHILDREN?

The most prevalent issue among children is dental cavities. Cavities are the most common dental problem experienced by children.

WHAT CAN I DO IF MY CHILD HAS A DENTAL EMERGENCY?

In the case of a dental emergency, it is important to assess the situation and act accordingly. If a tooth has been completely knocked out, contacting a dentist should be the first step. If possible, try to locate the tooth and handle it carefully. For a broken tooth, gather the fragments and allow the dentist to determine if they can be reattached. If no other options are available, clean the tooth and place it gently in the mouth, between the gum and the cheek. It is advisable to reach out to your dentist or a dental office for further guidance. It is crucial to avoid attempting DIY solutions as they may worsen the situation.

Dental emergencies can involve various scenarios, such as avulsion (tooth knocked out) or tooth fractures. Regardless of the specific situation, contacting a dentist is essential. Additionally, check for any foreign objects or injuries to the lips and seek a medical professional for a tetanus shot, especially if the injury occurred in a contaminated environment like a garden or outdoor area.

Determining whether a child should go to a hospital or a dental clinic depends on the severity of the injury. If it involves a severe dental emergency such as a jaw fracture, it is best to visit a hospital where urgent surgical intervention can be provided. In such cases, a dental clinic may not have the necessary facilities. Additionally, if a tetanus injection is required, immediate medical attention at a hospital is recommended. In some cases, patients have arrived at a dental clinic with initial dental emergencies like a fractured tooth, even during late hours. If the situation is not life-threatening, a dental clinic can be a suitable option.

However, for severe jaw fractures or emergencies that require immediate comprehensive care, it is advisable to go to an emergency room (ER) where a dentist can be contacted for specialized assistance. This ensures that all aspects, including mental and physical well-being, can be properly addressed in a timely manner.

Please note that the availability and setup of hospitals and dental clinics may vary by country or region. It is always recommended to follow the advice of healthcare professionals and seek appropriate medical attention based on the severity and nature of the dental emergency.

IS IT NECESSARY FOR MY CHILD TO HAVE DENTAL X-RAYS TAKEN?
X-rays are essential, especially for a child's first dental visit. They can reveal dental issues that may not be visible clinically, such as interdental cavities or abnormalities in tooth eruption. X-rays can also help identify missing or extra teeth that can impact the child's dental development. They provide valuable information about the bone structure and can help predict potential problems in the future. For example, a full mouth X-ray may show missing premolar tooth buds, indicating the need for future orthodontic treatment or implants.

In terms of safety, X-rays pose a minimal risk when done at appropriate intervals, such as once a year or every six months for larger scans like OPG. The digital X-rays are way safer than the traditional ones. The radiation exposure is lower than what you encounter during airport travel, and precautions such as lead aprons and thyroid shields are used to protect the patient. Additionally, digital X-rays have further reduced radiation exposure. For smaller X-rays like periapical scans, the radiation is negligible. Overall, the benefits of X-rays outweigh the potential risks when used responsibly. However, it is generally advisable to avoid X-rays for children below 2 years old unless absolutely necessary.

WHAT IS THE BEST WAY TO TREAT A CHILD'S CAVITIES?

Dental cavities in children can be managed in different ways depending on their cooperation. Ideally, the cavity should be cleaned and filled. If the cavity is deep but the pulp is not exposed, a layer of calcium hydroxide is applied before the filling. However, if the child is uncooperative, silver diamine fluoride (SDF) can be used to arrest the progression of the cavities and prevent them from reaching the pulp. While SDF may cause black discolouration, it is a safer alternative compared to the harmful effects of untreated cavities. When choosing the material for restoration, silver fillings are no longer practiced.

The options are between white fillings and crowns. Class two cavities, particularly those located between the teeth, are prone to fracture with fillings. In such cases, a crown is recommended for a more reliable and sealed restoration. However, the choice ultimately depends on the parents' preference. Some may prefer white fillings to maintain aesthetics, while others may opt for crowns for enhanced durability and cavity prevention. Regular check-ups and X-rays are crucial to detect any secondary decay or microleakage beneath the fillings. It is important to note that the choice of material and treatment approach should be based on professional evaluation and discussion with the dentist, taking into consideration the specific needs of the child and the extent of the cavities.

WHAT IS DENTAL SEALANT, AND IS IT NECESSARY FOR MY CHILD?

Our teeth, particularly the back teeth, have deep fissures that are difficult to clean effectively with brushing alone. These fissures are microscopic and not easily visible to the naked eye. Even thorough brushing cannot guarantee their cleanliness. However, with the use of dental sealants, we can make these rough and deep fissures smoother, creating a self-cleansing area. This provides relief during brushing and rinsing, knowing that nothing is getting trapped in those hard-to-reach areas. The accumulation of debris in these fissures is a common starting point for cavities in the first permanent molars, which are particularly vulnerable as they are still undergoing mineralization after the eruption. By sealing these fissures, we ensure that the bacteria have fewer hiding spots and reduce the risk of cavities in these vulnerable areas.

Sealants can sometimes become fractured. It is important to have regular follow-up visits with your dentist, especially a paediatric dentist, every 6 months. During these visits, the dentist will check the condition of the sealants. Factors such as eating habits and diet can influence the longevity of sealants. If they are no longer in place, they can be easily replaced. Redoing the sealants when necessary is the best approach to maintain their effectiveness.

WHAT ARE THE BENEFITS OF ORTHODONTIC TREATMENT FOR CHILDREN?
When considering orthodontic treatment for children, it is important to note that the benefits are more pronounced during the growing age. Starting treatment earlier can lead to reduced chances of relapse and improved confidence due to significant improvements in their smile. Additionally, orthodontic treatment at an early age can positively impact the shape and structure of the face, resulting in enhanced facial aesthetics. By initiating orthodontic treatment early, less invasive, lengthy, and complicated procedures may be avoided in the future. It allows for the natural growth stage to be

guided, without the need for excessive interventions. However, it is essential to direct the growth rather than stimulate or manipulate it extensively.

Regarding the cost of treatment, it can vary depending on various factors such as location and the specific dentist. While it is difficult to guarantee affordability, the long-term benefits, reduced complications, improved psychological well-being, and confidence make early orthodontic treatment a favourable option. The exact age to start orthodontic treatment varies on an individual basis and should be determined through consultation with a qualified dentist or orthodontist.

IS IT OKAY FOR MY CHILD TO PLAY SPORTS WITH BRACES?

The use of mouthguards can provide a solution for the situation, allowing for continued activities without significant restrictions. While it is important to exercise extra caution and take additional care, the availability of mouthguards helps in safeguarding the braces. The mouthguard can be custom-made to accommodate the presence of braces, ensuring a proper fit and adequate protection.

WHAT ARE THE RISKS OF NOT TREATING MY CHILD'S CAVITIES?

Neglecting the treatment of cavities can have serious consequences. If cavities are left untreated, they can progress to the point where they affect the pulp of the tooth, leading to pain and discomfort. Although some children with milk teeth may not experience immediate pain due to less developed nerves, the damage can still worsen. Without intervention, there is a risk of developing gum swelling, extraoral swelling, and even nighttime pain, causing significant discomfort for the child. In severe cases, the tooth may be so extensively damaged internally that extraction becomes necessary.

Occasionally, swelling could be big enough to even pose a life threatening situation by blocking the airway pipe. Avoiding prompt treatment can result in tooth loss and additional financial expenses, such as requiring a root canal treatment or even undergoing general anesthesia if the child is uncooperative. It is always better to address dental issues earlier to prevent more extensive and costly treatments later on.

HOW CAN I PREVENT BABY BOTTLE TOOTH DECAY IN MY CHILD?

The prevention of baby bottle tooth decay begins with avoiding the introduction of milk bottles to infants. It is not necessary for a child to consume milk exclusively from a bottle. Instead, small silicon soup spoons or cups can be used for feeding. This helps prevent prolonged exposure to milk and the habit of holding the bottle for extended periods, especially while lying down. When milk is continuously consumed from a bottle, the acid levels in the mouth remain high, leading to tooth erosion and cavities. By encouraging children to sit upright and finish their milk in one sitting and a definite duration, the risk of baby bottle tooth decay can be minimized.

This also helps instill proper eating habits, emphasizing the importance of completing meals promptly rather than treating them as a pastime. After feeding, it is essential to clean the teeth and encourage rinsing. Brushing should be performed either by the parent or by the child, depending on their age. It is crucial to wean children from the bottle at the appropriate age, as both pacifiers and milk bottles can impact dental health and jaw growth. By limiting prolonged bottle use, parents can promote healthier teeth and overall oral development.

Regarding milk's effect on teeth, while milk does provide essential nutrients like calcium and phosphorus, it also contains natural sugars. When milk is consumed continuously, the sugar in it contributes to the formation of dental decay. It is important to avoid allowing milk to remain in the mouth for prolonged periods, as this can lead to the growth of bacteria and plaque, resulting in tooth decay. It is recommended to provide alternative sources of calcium and minerals through dental-friendly products like tooth mousse or fluoride supplements, which focus solely on delivering the necessary minerals without the added sugar found in milk.

HOW CAN I FIND A PAEDIATRIC DENTIST FOR MY CHILD?

From my perspective, a good paediatric dentist should possess qualities such as compassion, patience, and the ability to connect with children. They should be willing to meet the children at their level, befriend them, and maintain a playful demeanour. Kindness and empathy are crucial in creating a comfortable and positive dental experience for young patients. It is also important for paediatric dentists to have a thorough understanding of their field and possess the necessary knowledge and expertise.

Furthermore, patience is of utmost importance as paediatric dentists must not only engage with the child but also effectively communicate with their parents or caregivers. The ability to manage both the child and their parents is a key aspect of providing quality paediatric dental care. One can refer to online reviews or go by the word of mouth from you're acquaintance regarding a Pediatric Dentist.

HOW CAN I HELP MY CHILD MAINTAIN GOOD ORAL HYGIENE WHILE WEARING APPLIANCES?

When using removable appliances, it is important to maintain proper hygiene. Avoid wearing them while eating or consuming anything. Regular cleaning is necessary, especially focusing on the areas that come into contact with oral tissues. This includes regular brushing, flossing, and tongue cleaning. Depending on the type of appliance, interdental toothbrushes and fluoride toothpaste can be used. Nano hydroxyapatite toothpaste is also available as an alternative for those who prefer fluoride-free options. Regular professional cleanings are highly recommended as appliances require specialized care that cannot be achieved at home alone. Additionally, fluoride varnish treatments can contribute to maintaining good oral hygiene. Alongside hygiene practices, a fibrous diet can help keep the teeth surfaces clean.

For children with appliances or braces, frequent dental visits are necessary. It is advisable to visit the dentist every three months to ensure proper maintenance and address any potential issues promptly. In some cases, even more frequent visits may be required, as individual needs may vary. By attending regular dental check-ups, the child's oral health can be effectively monitored and any necessary adjustments or cleanings can be performed in a timely manner. Please note that the recommended frequency of dental visits may vary depending on the specific circumstances and the dentist's professional judgment. It is always best to consult with a dental professional for personalized advice and guidance.

10.6 - FEAR/PAIN

by Dr. PRRIYA PORWAL FROM UNITED ARAB EMIRATES

IS SEDATION DENTISTRY NECESSARY FOR CHILDREN?

The decision to pursue sedation for dental treatment is not a new concept. It is an option that can be considered if it is deemed necessary for a child's specific needs. It is important not to overlook oral hygiene or oral health simply because a child may be uncooperative. However, it is crucial to acknowledge that sedation does come with inherent risks. In the UAE, inhalation sedation is the only form of sedation permitted in dental clinics. Any other type of sedation requires the presence of an anesthesiologist and must be performed in a hospital setting. Initially, inhalation sedation is attempted in the dental clinic. If a child remains uncooperative even with this method, intravenous (IV) sedation becomes an alternative. IV sedation is administered in a hospital operating room under the supervision of an anesthesiologist.

In cases where a child has multiple cavities and is uncooperative, full mouth rehabilitation under general anesthesia may be recommended. It is important to explain to parents or guardians that this treatment is necessary. By following proper protocols and adhering to the instructions provided by the anesthesiologist during the pre-surgical phase, the risks associated with anesthesia can be minimized. Following guidelines such as fasting for the appropriate duration before the procedure helps ensure the safety of the child. The decision to proceed with sedation should be made in consultation with a dental professional and anesthesiologist, taking into consideration the specific circumstances and needs of the child.

HOW CAN I HELP MY CHILD COPE WITH TOOTH LOSS?

When children face the prospect of losing a tooth, it can often lead to psychological distress. Since years, Tooth-fairy has been coming to the rescue though. It is not uncommon for kids to experience pain and anxiety due to the thought of losing their teeth. As dental professionals, it becomes important to reassure and educate them about the reasons behind tooth extraction and the benefits it will bring. Additionally, we can provide solutions to address the concerns they may have about the empty space left behind.

One approach is to offer a functional space maintainer, which not only serves its purpose but also has an aesthetic appearance. This appliance can fill the gap, providing a temporary solution while assuring the child that the missing tooth will be replaced naturally in due time. To further alleviate their worries, we can show them the X-ray and explain the growth process, giving them hope and reassurance that new teeth will emerge. It is crucial to approach this situation with empathy and understanding, helping children navigate the emotional aspect of losing a tooth.

HOW CAN I RELIEVE MY CHILD'S TOOTH ERUPTION PAIN?

To alleviate teething discomfort in children, there are various options available. One approach is to use teething gels, which can be recommended by your dentist. There are several types of gels on the market that can provide relief. Another natural remedy is to allow them to bite on something cold, such as a chilled carrot or a teething ring that has been placed in the freezer. The cold sensation can help soothe the gums and improve eruption. For those who prefer non-medicated options, homeopathic remedies may be considered. Some individuals find relief using ice or cold fermentation techniques.

In the case of toddlers or young children, frozen teething rings can be used to provide relief and comfort. In more severe cases of teething pain, especially when permanent molars are erupting, a painkiller may be recommended. However, it is important to consult with a healthcare professional before administering any medication to ensure proper dosage and suitability for the child's age and condition.

WHAT ARE THE RISKS OF USING TEETHING GELS AND CREAMS?

The frequency of use for teething remedies depends on the specific ingredients and their concentrations. It is important to follow the guidance of your dentist, doctor, or physician regarding the proper usage. However, it is generally not recommended to use medicated teething remedies with ingredients like lignocaine too frequently. Natural remedies may have different recommendations. In cases of severe teething discomfort, it may be necessary to provide a painkiller under the guidance of a healthcare professional.

Alternatively, offering teething rings or allowing them to bite on cold vegetables or fruits can provide relief, particularly for toddlers. It is crucial to prioritize the safety and well-being of the child and consult with healthcare professionals for appropriate guidance on the use of teething remedies.

HOW CAN I HELP MY CHILD RECOVER AFTER A DENTAL PROCEDURE?

During dental procedures involving local anesthesia, it is important to take certain precautions to ensure the child's comfort and prevent complications. Firstly, it is crucial to ensure that the child does not bite their lips or cheeks, as this can lead to ulcers, causing additional distress for parents. Care should be taken to prevent any strenuous activities or heavy exertion immediately after an extraction to minimize the risk of bleeding. Using a straw should be avoided as it can create negative pressure in the mouth and disrupt the clotting process. It is also advised to refrain from consuming hot, spicy, or carbonated drinks, as they may cause discomfort or interfere with the healing process.

If necessary, the dentist may recommend a painkiller to manage any post-procedure pain, ensuring a more positive experience. Lastly, it is important to emphasize to the child that they should not skip brushing their teeth, even after an extraction, to maintain good oral hygiene.

Please note that these guidelines are provided as general information and it is always best to follow the specific instructions and advice given by the dentist for each individual case.

10.7 - MONEY

by Dr. PRRIYA PORWAL FROM UNITED ARAB EMIRATES

WHAT IS THE COST OF PAEDIATRIC DENTAL CARE?

The cost of dental treatments for children compared to adults can vary depending on several factors, including the specific treatment needed and the insurance coverage. It is important to note that cost may differ between different healthcare systems and regions. To determine the exact cost, it is advisable to consult with a dental professional or contact local dental clinics to inquire about the pricing and any insurance coverage available for paediatric dental care.

ARE THOSE COVERED BY THE GOVERNMENT?

In Abu Dhabi, the government provides insurance coverage for Emiratis, offering them a privileged healthcare system. Emiratis in Abu Dhabi enjoy comprehensive coverage for almost all treatments, with government insurance taking care of the expenses. However, it's important to note that the coverage may vary between different Emirates. For instance, in Dubai, locals are required to pay twenty percent of the treatment cost, as preventive procedures may not be fully covered by insurance. This means that Abu Dhabi locals have a higher level of privilege when it comes to healthcare coverage. It's essential to check the specific insurance policies and coverage details based on the Emirates and individual circumstances.

ARE INSURANCE COVERING CHILD DENTAL CARE?

Unfortunately, not all private insurance plans provide comprehensive coverage for children's dental care. Some insurance plans may have limited coverage with low caps, such as a maximum coverage limit of around two thousand dirhams. Additionally, not all insurance plans include specific coverage for paediatric dental care but rather offer general dental coverage for all ages. It's important to carefully review the terms and conditions of each insurance plan to determine the extent of coverage for children's dental care.

10.8 - HABITS

by Dr. PRRIYA PORWAL FROM UNITED ARAB EMIRATES

IS THUMB-SUCKING HARMFUL TO MY CHILD'S TEETH?

Thumb sucking can have detrimental effects on a child's oral health and development. Firstly, it can create a psychological dependency on the habit, making it difficult for the child to break the habit as they grow older. Secondly, it can impact the growth of the jaw, leading to changes in the shape of the palate and facial structure. This can result in an elongated face and misalignment of the teeth. Furthermore, prolonged thumb sucking can cause the teeth to protrude, making them more susceptible to injuries. As mentioned before, it's important to be aware of these potential harms and take steps to discourage thumb-sucking in order to promote healthy dental and jaw development for your child.

HOW CAN I ENCOURAGE MY CHILD TO STOP THUMB-SUCKING?

Thumb sucking should ideally be stopped by the age of four. If the habit is discontinued by this age, the adverse effects can be reversible as the jaw growth is still in a dynamic process. When thumb sucking is ceased, the pressure from the lips can guide the teeth and bone to develop in a proper alignment. This ensures that the permanent teeth erupt in a straight manner, without the issues observed in the primary dentition. Therefore, the age of four is considered the best and ideal time to address and eliminate the thumb-sucking habit.

If simple techniques and gentle methods do not prove effective in stopping thumb sucking by this age, it may be necessary to adopt more assertive measures. Thumb-sucking deterrent devices, such as thumb guards or application of bitter edible material on thumb, can be used. There are also appliances available that create discomfort when the child attempts to engage in thumb-sucking, serving as a deterrent. For example, some appliances have a roller placed on the palate, allowing the child to play with it but not obtain the same pleasure as thumb-sucking.

Over time, the hope is that the child will cease the habit. It is important to address thumb sucking as early as possible to prevent long-term oral and dental complications. By discontinuing the habit at an appropriate age, the child's dental and jaw development can proceed in a healthier and more desirable manner.

HOW CAN I PREVENT MY CHILD FROM GRINDING THEIR TEETH AT NIGHT?

Grinding of teeth, also known as bruxism, can occur due to various reasons such as stress, intestinal worms, or even nightmares. Identifying the underlying cause is crucial in addressing the issue effectively. Once the cause is determined, appropriate measures can be taken to alleviate the grinding and its potential effects. One common method of preventing the damage caused by teeth grinding is through the use of night guards. Night guards are custom-made, flexible plastic devices that are designed to fit your child's teeth. They are typically worn on one arch of the mouth and act as a protective barrier, preventing the teeth from grinding against each other.

It is important to consult with a dental professional to diagnose the root cause of teeth grinding and to ensure the night guard is fitted properly for optimal protection. They can provide further guidance on managing the underlying cause and offer recommendations tailored to your child's specific situation.

WHAT ARE THE DANGERS OF SHARING UTENSILS AND DRINKS WITH MY CHILD?

Sharing utensils and drinks may seem like a loving gesture, but it can also lead to the transfer of bacteria. It's important to understand that when you share utensils or engage in activities like kissing on the lips, you are not just sharing love but potentially harmful bacteria as well. While you may not feel the immediate impact, your child may experience its consequences later on. As a dental professional, I always advise parents to refrain from kissing their children on the lips. This is because the act of kissing can transfer bacteria that may contribute to oral health issues.

Additionally, it's crucial to avoid sharing utensils, even among siblings. For instance, if one sibling has cavities or dental problems while the other is still in the process of tooth eruption, sharing utensils can expose the younger sibling's teeth to harmful bacteria from the elder sibling.

Sharing and caring are wonderful qualities, but when it comes to oral health, it's best to prioritize hygiene and prevent the spread of bacteria. Encouraging good oral hygiene practices, such as using individual utensils and maintaining proper dental care, will help protect your child's oral health in the long run.

HOW CAN I HELP MY CHILD AVOID JAW PROBLEMS?

If your child is experiencing dental problems like cavities, teeth grinding, oral habits, or mouth breathing, there are various approaches to address each issue. However, it's important to note that these solutions should be determined and recommended by a qualified dental professional. For cavity-related concerns, your child can use toothpaste with fluoride before going to sleep. This can help strengthen the teeth and prevent further decay. It's crucial to follow the guidance provided by your dentist regarding the application of toothpaste. If It Is a skeletal relation or occlusion problem, a pediatric dentist or an orthdodontist can find you a solution.

HOW CAN I PREVENT DENTAL PROBLEMS IN MY CHILD WHILE THEY ARE SLEEPING?

When it comes to teeth grinding, wearing a night guard can be beneficial. A night guard is a customized, flexible plastic appliance that helps protect the teeth from grinding forces during sleep. Your dentist can evaluate your child's specific situation and recommend the appropriate night guard. For oral habits such as thumb sucking, the solutions may vary. As mentioned earlier, you can try using techniques like wearing a long-sleeve shirt or T-shirt to discourage thumb-sucking during sleep. However, if the habit persists, it's important to consult a paediatric dentist who can provide tailored appliances or other interventions to address the habit effectively.

In the case of mouth breathing, it's essential to determine the underlying cause. If it's related to anatomical issues like enlarged adenoids, an evaluation by an ENT specialist is necessary to address the root cause. If it's a habitual habit, your paediatric dentist can guide you on appropriate interventions and provide the necessary support. The best course of action is to seek professional advice from a dental specialist who can assess your child's specific needs and provide personalized recommendations and treatment options.

This is **ALPHA DENTISTRY vol. 3, PAEDIATRIC DENTISTRY FAQ**. Welcome to the Alphas.

Dr. BAK NGUYEN

CONCLUSION
by Dr. BAK NGUYEN

What a journey, 4 months of international cooperation to make Alpha 3 a success! I was barely out of the writing of Alpha 2 (implantology) we started this new endeavour. As said many times already, we, Alphas, are doing this to change the narrative of our profession and to be closer to the people, the general public, not just our patients.

I believe that promoting our profession requires more than just having a great personality. Sure, we all have great intentions and different personalities, but as I am writing this book with paedodontists, one fact has emerged without a doubt: paedodontists are the most humane dentists within our ranks.

In my personal opinion, if we are rebranding our profession, paedodontists should be at the forefront as ambassadors and our spokespeople! This came to light after I interviewed so many of our colleagues from different fields of dentistry. Paedondontists are not just kind and aware, but they have that core kindness to care about people first, teeth come much later.

A specific example that I can give on the matter is to the question of, why is it potentially harmful for an adult to share utensils and drink with a child, where every doctor would have said contamination, each of the paedodontists took the time to explain in length the cause and effect without ever mentioning the word contamination.

In other words, you care as much for the feelings of the person in front of you as you care for the science being shared. And because of that, the message has a much greater chance to reach its audience.

When I started our endeavour to democratize our science and to unify dentistry, communication was the only thing I had to build on. Well, I am so glad that by writing this series of books, we are starting to sort out the role of each specialty.

To make this work, we should act as a whole, not as a collective of individuals, all fighting to pass our message across. To clean the noise and to rectify our image and role, the intent should be straightforward and simple: to help people understand, so they can care. Thank you for being mindful of your words, of your patients and the people surrounding them.

"Even fear dissipates as communication is well-established since it allows trust to build."

Dr. Bak Nguyen

With 10 international co-authors from 7 different countries, 202 years of cumulative clinical experience, we, Dr. Paul Dominique, Dr. Aurora Alva, Dr. Richard Simpson, Dr. Nour Ammar, Dr. Marilyne Sandor, Dr. Nidhi Tajena, Dr. Pierluigi Pelagalli, Dr. Ailin Cabrera-Matta, Dr. Prriya Porwal, and myself, Dr. Bak Nguyen, from Germany, from Egypt, from Italy, from Peru, from the United Arab Emirates, from USA, from Canada, we give you **ALPHA DENTISTRY volume 3, PAEDIATRIC DENTISTRY FAQ.**

May this work be a step in a new direction, may it answer your questions and bring us closer together.

"I treat people, not teeth."

Dr. Bak Nguyen

Before closing this chapter, please allow me to especially thank Dr. Aurora Alva for being a pillar in the recruitment of this international cast. Dr. Paul Dominique, Dr. Richard Simpson, thank you for helping in the recruitment effort and in keeping the team as a cohesive unit. Our Alphas international organization is made possible thanks to your effort.

That said, I will thank each and every one of you, Marilyne, Nidhi, Prriya, Nour, Ailin, Aurora, Pierluigi, Richard, Paul to have accepted my invitation and joined me in the democratization and unification of dentistry. I am humbled and privileged to serve with you, my colleagues, my friends.

This is **ALPHA DENTISTRY vol. 3, PAEDIATRIC DENTISTRY FAQ**. Welcome to the Alphas.

Dr. BAK NGUYEN

ANNEX

GLOSSARY OF Dr. BAK's LIBRARY

1

1SELF -080

REINVENT YOURSELF FROM ANY CRISIS

BY Dr. BAK NGUYEN

1SELF is about reinventing yourself to rise from any crisis. Written in the midst of the COVID war, now more than ever, we need hope and the know-how to bridge the future. More than just the journey of Dr. Bak, this time, Dr. Bak is sharing his journey with mentors and people who built part of the world as we know it. Interviewed in this book, CHRISTIAN TRUDEAU, former CEO and FOUNDER of BCE EMERGIS (BELL CANADA), he also digitalized the Montreal Stock Exchange. RON KLEIN, American Innovator, inventor of the magnetic stripe of the credit card, of MLS (Multi-listing services) and the man who digitalized WALL STREET bonds markets. ANDRE CHATELAIN, former first vice-president of the MOVEMENT DESJARDINS. Dr. JEAN DE SERRES, former CEO of HEMA QUEBEC. These men created billions in values and have changed our lives, even without us knowing. They all come together to share their experiences and knowledge to empower each and everyone to emerge stronger from this crisis, from any crisis.

A

AFTERMATH -063
BUSINESS AFTER THE GREAT PAUSE
BY Dr. BAK NGUYEN & Dr. ERIC LACOSTE

In AFTERMATH, Dr. Bak joins forces with Community leader and philanthrope Dr. Eric Lacoste. Two powerful minds and forces of nature in the reaction to the worst economic meltdown in modern times. We are all victims of the CORONA virus. Both just like humans have learnt to adapt to survive, so is our economy. Most business structures and management philosophies are inherited from the age of industrialization and beyond. COVID-19 has shot down the world economy for months. At the time of the AFTERMATH, the truth is many corporations and organizations will either have to upgrade to the INFORMATION AGE or disappear. More than the INFORMATION upgrade, the era of SOCIAL MEDIA and the MILLENNIALS are driving a revolution in the core philosophy of all organizations. Profit is not king anymore, support is. In this time and age where a teenager with a social account can compete with the million dollars PR firm, social implication is now the new cornerstone. Those who will adapt will prevail and prosper, while the resistance and old guards will soon be forgotten as fossils of a past era.

ALPHA DENTISTRY vol. 1 -104
DIGITAL ORTHODONTIC FAQ
BY Dr. BAK NGUYEN

In ALPHA DENTISTRY, DIGITAL ORTHODONTICS FAQ, Dr. Bak is looking to democratize the science of dentistry, starting with orthodontics. In a word, he is sharing everything a patient needs to know on the matter in FAQ form. In order to make the knowledge complete and universal, Dr. Bak has invited Alpha Dentists from all around the world to join in and answer the same question. With Alpha Dentists from America and Europe, ALPHA DENTISTRY is the first effort to create a universal knowledge in the field of dentistry, starting with orthodontics. ALPHA DENTISTRY, DIGITAL ORTHODONTICS FAQ is in response to the COVID crisis, the shortage of staff crisis, and the effort to unify dentistry to the Information Age, as discussed in RELEVANCY and COVIDCONOMICS, THE DENTAL INDUSTRY.

ALPHA DENTISTRY vol. 1 -109
DIGITAL ORTHODONTIC FAQ ASSEMBLED EDITION

CANADA GERMANY INDIA USA SPAIN

BY Dr. BAK NGUYEN, Dr. PAUL OUELLETTE, Dr. PAUL DOMINIQUE, Dr. MARIA KUNSTADTER, Dr. EDWARD J. ZUCKERBERG, Dr. MASHA KHAGHANI, Dr. SUJATA BASAWARAJ, Dr. ALVA AURORA, Dr. JUDITH BÄUMLER, and Dr. ASHISH GUPTA

In ALPHA DENTISTRY, DIGITAL ORTHODONTICS FAQ, Dr. Bak is democratizing the science of dentistry, starting with orthodontics. In a word, he is sharing everything a patient needs to know on the matter in FAQ form, simple words you'll understand.10 International Alpha Doctors, from USA, Spain, Germany, India, and Canada are joining forces to make the knowledge complete and universal. ALPHA DENTISTRY is the first effort to create a universal knowledge in the field of dentistry, this is the orthodontics volume. This is the most ambitious book project in the History of Dentistry. ALPHA DENTISTRY is in response to the COVID crisis, the shortage of staff crisis, and the effort to unify dentistry to the Information Age, as discussed in RELEVANCY and COVIDCONOMICS, THE DENTAL INDUSTRY.

ALPHA DENTISTRY vol. 1 -113
DIGITAL ORTHODONTIC FAQ INTERNATIONAL EDITION

ENGLISH FRENCH GERMAN HINDI SPANISH

BY Dr. BAK NGUYEN, Dr. PAUL OUELLETTE, Dr. PAUL DOMINIQUE, Dr. MARIA KUNSTADTER, Dr. EDWARD J. ZUCKERBERG, Dr. MASHA KHAGHANI, Dr. SUJATA BASAWARAJ, Dr. ALVA AURORA, Dr. JUDITH BÄUMLER, and Dr. ASHISH GUPTA

In ALPHA DENTISTRY, DIGITAL ORTHODONTICS FAQ, Dr. Bak is democratizing the science of dentistry, starting with orthodontics. In a word, he is sharing everything a patient needs to know on the matter in FAQ form, simple words you'll understand.10 International Alpha Doctors, from USA, Spain, Germany, India, and Canada are joining forces to make the knowledge complete and universal. ALPHA DENTISTRY is the first effort to create a universal knowledge in the field of dentistry, this is the orthodontics volume. This is the most ambitious book project in the History of Dentistry. ALPHA DENTISTRY is in response to the COVID crisis, the shortage of staff crisis, and the effort to unify dentistry to the Information Age, as discussed in RELEVANCY and COVIDCONOMICS, THE DENTAL INDUSTRY.

ALPHA DENTISTRY vol. 2 -127
IMPLANTOLOGY FAQ ASSEMBLED EDITION

ALBANIA BRAZIL CANADA INDIA MALAYSIA PORTUGAL SPAIN USA
BY Dr. BAK NGUYEN, Dr. ERIC LACOSTE , Dr. PRETINDER SINGH, Dr. SANDEEP SINGH, Dr. ERIC PULVER, Dr. ARASH HAKHAMIAN, Dr. MAHSA KHAGHANI, Dr. BENNETE FERNANDES, Dr. RAQUEL ZITA GOMES, Dr. SANDRA FABIANO and Dr. GURIEN DEMIRAQI

In ALPHA DENTISTRY, IMPLANTOLOGY FAQ, Dr. Bak is democratizing the science of dentistry, with the sub-specialty of IMPLANTOLOGY, which expertise is shared between Periodontists, Oral Surgeons and Dentists. In a word, he is sharing everything a patient needs to know on the matter in FAQ form, simple words you'll understand.11 International Alpha Doctors, from USA, India, Portugal, Spain, Brazil, Malaysia, Albania and Canada are joining forces to make the knowledge complete and universal. ALPHA DENTISTRY is the first effort to create a universal knowledge in the field of dentistry, this is the IMPLANTOLOGY volume. This is the most ambitious book project in the History of Dentistry. The whole book is covered in English and each author with a different native tongue is also covering their chapters in their native language. ALPHA DENTISTRY is in response to the COVID crisis, the shortage of staff crisis, and the effort to unify dentistry to the Information Age, as discussed in RELEVANCY and COVIDCONOMICS, THE DENTAL INDUSTRY.

ALPHA DENTISTRY vol. 2 -128
IMPLANTOLOGY FAQ INTERNATIONAL EDITION

ALBANIAN ENGLISH FRANÇAIS GERMAN HINDI ITALIAN KANNADA MALAY MANDARIN PORTUGUESE SPANISH
BY Dr. BAK NGUYEN, Dr. ERIC LACOSTE , Dr. PRETINDER SINGH, Dr. SANDEEP SINGH, Dr. ERIC PULVER, Dr. ARASH HAKHAMIAN, Dr. MAHSA KHAGHANI, Dr. BENNETE FERNANDES, Dr. RAQUEL ZITA GOMES, Dr. SANDRA FABIANO and Dr. GURIEN DEMIRAQI

In ALPHA DENTISTRY, IMPLANTOLOGY FAQ, Dr. Bak is democratizing the science of dentistry, with the sub-specialty of IMPLANTOLOGY, which expertise is shared between Periodontists, Oral Surgeons and Dentists. In a word, he is sharing everything a patient needs to know on the matter in FAQ form, simple words you'll understand.11 International Alpha Doctors, from USA, India, Portugal, Spain, Brazil, Malaysia, Albania and Canada are joining forces to make the knowledge complete and universal. ALPHA DENTISTRY is the first effort to create a universal knowledge in the field of dentistry, this is the IMPLANTOLOGY volume. This is the most ambitious book project in the History of Dentistry. The whole book is covered in English and each author with a different native tongue is also covering their chapters in their native language. ALPHA DENTISTRY is in response to the COVID crisis, the shortage of staff crisis, and the effort to unify dentistry to the Information Age, as discussed in RELEVANCY and COVIDCONOMICS, THE DENTAL INDUSTRY.

ALPHA DENTISTRY vol. 3 -131
PAEDIATRIC FAQ ASSEMBLED EDITION

🇨🇦 CANADA 🇪🇬 EGYPT 🇩🇪 GERMANY 🇮🇹 ITALY 🇵🇪 PERU 🇦🇪 UNITED ARAB EMIRATES 🇺🇸 USA

BY Dr. BAK NGUYEN, Dr. PAUL DOMINIQUE, Dr. RICHARD SIMPSON, Dr. MARILYNE SANDOR, Dr. AURORA ALVA, Dr. NOUR AMMAR, Dr. AILIN CABRERA-MATTA, Dr. NIDHI TANEJA, Dr. PRRIYA PORWAL, and Dr. PIERLUIGI PELAGALLI

In ALPHA DENTISTRY, PAEDIATRIC FAQ, Dr. Bak is democratizing the science of dentistry, this time, focusing on children. From all of dentistry, this is the kindest and most humane specialty of DENTISTRY. From the USA to Germany, Peru to Egypt and Canada, experts around the world are joining this collaborative effort welcome, reassure, and empower parents and kids on their quest to a healthy mouth. ALPHA DENTISTRY is the first effort to create a universal knowledge in the field of dentistry, this is the PAEDIATRIC volume. This is the most ambitious book project in the History of Dentistry. The whole book is covered in English and each author with a different native tongue is also covering their chapters in their native language. ALPHA DENTISTRY is in response to the COVID crisis, the shortage of staff crisis, and the effort to unify dentistry to the Information Age, as discussed in RELEVANCY and COVIDCONOMICS, THE DENTAL INDUSTRY.

ALPHA DENTISTRY vol. 3 -132
PAEDIATRIC FAQ INTERNATIONAL EDITION

🇺🇸 ENGLISH 🇪🇬 ARABIC 🇨🇦 FRANÇAIS 🇮🇹 ITALIAN 🇵🇪 SPANISH

BY Dr. BAK NGUYEN, Dr. PAUL DOMINIQUE, Dr. RICHARD SIMPSON, Dr. MARILYNE SANDOR, Dr. AURORA ALVA, Dr. NOUR AMMAR, Dr. AILIN CABRERA-MATTA, Dr. NIDHI TANEJA, Dr. PRRIYA PORWAL, and Dr. PIERLUIGI PELAGALLI

In ALPHA DENTISTRY, PAEDIATRIC FAQ, Dr. Bak is democratizing the science of dentistry, this time, focusing on children. From all of dentistry, this is the kindest and most humane specialty of DENTISTRY. From the USA to Germany, Peru to Egypt and Canada, experts around the world are joining this collaborative effort welcome, reassure, and empower parents and kids on their quest to a healthy mouth. ALPHA DENTISTRY is the first effort to create a universal knowledge in the field of dentistry, this is the PAEDIATRIC volume. This is the most ambitious book project in the History of Dentistry. The whole book is covered in English and each author with a different native tongue is also covering their chapters in their native language. ALPHA DENTISTRY is in response to the COVID crisis, the shortage of staff crisis, and the effort to unify dentistry to the Information Age, as discussed in RELEVANCY and COVIDCONOMICS, THE DENTAL INDUSTRY.

ALPHA DENTISTRY vol. 4 -139
PAEDIATRIC DENTISTRY FAQ ASSEMBLED EDITION

🏴 ALBANIA 🏴 AUSTRALIA 🇨🇦 CANADA 🏴 GERMANY 🏴 INDIA 🏴 IRAN 🏴 MALAYSIA 🏴 SPAIN 🏴 USA

BY Dr. BAK NGUYEN, Dr. ERIC LACOSTE, Dr. MAZIAR SHAHZAD DOWLATSHAHI, Dr. BENNETE FERNANDES, Dr. MEENU BHASIN, Dr. HASTEE BHANUSHALI, Dr. ROBERT M. PICK, Dr. AMIN MOTAMEDI, Dr. TIHANA DIVNIC-RESNIK, Dr. ARNE VON STERNHEIM, Dr. FERNANDO ARPÓN MORENO and Dr. GURIEN DEMIRAQI

In ALPHA DENTISTRY, PERIODONTICS FAQ, Dr. Bak is democratizing the science of dentistry, with the sub-specialty of PERIODONTOLOGY, which expertise is shared between Periodontists, Oral Surgeons and Dentists. In a word, he is sharing everything a patient needs to know on the matter in FAQ form, simple words you'll understand.11 International Alpha Doctors, from the USA, India, Australia, Iran, Malaysia, Albania and Canada are joining forces to make the knowledge complete and universal. ALPHA DENTISTRY is the first effort to create a universal knowledge in the field of dentistry, this is the PERIODONTICS volume. This is the most ambitious book project in the History of Dentistry. The whole book is covered in English and each author with a different native tongue is also covering their chapters in their native language. ALPHA DENTISTRY is in response to the COVID crisis, the shortage of staff crisis, and the effort to unify dentistry to the Information Age, as discussed in RELEVANCY and COVIDCONOMICS, THE DENTAL INDUSTRY.

ALPHA DENTISTRY vol. 4 -140
PAEDIATRIC DENTISTRY FAQ INTERNATIONAL EDITION

🏴 ENGLISH 🇨🇦 FRENCH 🏴 GERMAN 🏴 HINDI 🇮🇹 ITALIAN 🏴 MANDARIN 🏴 MALAY 🏴 ARABIC 🏴 SPANISH 🏴 SHQIP

BY Dr. BAK NGUYEN, Dr. ERIC LACOSTE, Dr. MAZIAR SHAHZAD DOWLATSHAHI, Dr. BENNETE FERNANDES, Dr. MEENU BHASIN, Dr. HASTEE BHANUSHALI, Dr. ROBERT M. PICK, Dr. AMIN MOTAMEDI, Dr. TIHANA DIVNIC-RESNIK, Dr. ARNE VON STERNHEIM, Dr. FERNANDO ARPÓN MORENO and Dr. GURIEN DEMIRAQI

In ALPHA DENTISTRY, PERIODONTICS FAQ, Dr. Bak is democratizing the science of dentistry, with the sub-specialty of PERIODONTOLOGY, which expertise is shared between Periodontists, Oral Surgeons and Dentists. In a word, he is sharing everything a patient needs to know on the matter in FAQ form, simple words you'll understand.11 International Alpha Doctors, from the USA, India, Germany, Spain, Australia, Iran, Malaysia, Albania and Canada are joining forces to make the knowledge complete and universal. ALPHA DENTISTRY is the first effort to create a universal knowledge in the field of dentistry, this is the PERIODONTICS volume. This is the most ambitious book project in the History of Dentistry. The whole book is covered in English and each author with a different native tongue is also covering their chapters in their native language. ALPHA DENTISTRY is in response to the COVID crisis, the shortage of staff crisis, and the effort to unify dentistry to the Information Age, as discussed in RELEVANCY and COVIDCONOMICS, THE DENTAL INDUSTRY.

ALPHA DENTISTRY vol. 5 141
PAEDIATRIC DENTISTRY FAQ ASSEMBLED EDITION

AUSTRALIA CANADA FRANCE LITHUANIA PERU TURKEY UKRAINE USA
BY Dr. BAK NGUYEN, Dr. JULIO REYNAFARJE, Dr. LINA DUSEVIČIŪTĖ, Dr. NAZARIY MYKHAYLYUK, Dr. CLAUDE MOUAFO, Dr. MANOJ RAJAN, Dr. LOUIS KAUFMAN, Dr. LILIAN SHI and Dr. YASEMIN OZKAN

In ALPHA DENTISTRY, COSMETIC DENTISTRY FAQ, Dr. Bak is democratizing the science of dentistry, with the sub specialty of COSMETIC DENTISTRY, which expertise is shared between Prosthodontists and Dentists. In a word, he is sharing everything a patient needs to know on the matter in FAQ form, simple words you'll understand. International Alpha Doctors, from the USA, France, Peru, Lithuania, Ukraine, Australia, Turkey and Canada are joining forces to make the knowledge complete and universal. ALPHA DENTISTRY is the first effort to create a universal knowledge in the field of dentistry, this is the COSMETIC DENTISTRY volume. This is the most ambitious book project in the History of Dentistry. The whole book is covered in English and each author with a different native tongue is also covering their chapters in their native language. ALPHA DENTISTRY is in response to the COVID crisis, the shortage of staff crisis, and the effort to unify dentistry to the Information Age, as discussed in RELEVANCY and COVIDCONOMICS, THE DENTAL INDUSTRY.

ALPHA DENTISTRY vol. 5 142
PAEDIATRIC DENTISTRY FAQ INTERNATIONAL EDITION

ENGLISH ARABIC FRENCH LITHUANIAN SPANISH UKRAINIAN
BY Dr. BAK NGUYEN, Dr. JULIO REYNAFARJE, Dr. LINA DUSEVIČIŪTĖ, Dr. NAZARIY MYKHAYLYUK, Dr. CLAUDE MOUAFO, Dr. MANOJ RAJAN, Dr. LOUIS KAUFMAN, Dr. LILIAN SHI and Dr. YASEMIN OZKAN

In ALPHA DENTISTRY, COSMETIC DENTISTRY FAQ, Dr. Bak is democratizing the science of dentistry, with the sub specialty of COSMETIC DENTISTRY, which expertise is shared between Prosthodontists and Dentists. In a word, he is sharing everything a patient needs to know on the matter in FAQ form, simple words you'll understand. International Alpha Doctors, from the USA, France, Peru, Lithuania, Ukraine, Australia, Turkey and Canada are joining forces to make the knowledge complete and universal. ALPHA DENTISTRY is the first effort to create a universal knowledge in the field of dentistry, this is the COSMETIC DENTISTRY volume. This is the most ambitious book project in the History of Dentistry. The whole book is covered in English and each author with a different native tongue is also covering their chapters in their native language. ALPHA DENTISTRY is in response to the COVID crisis, the shortage of staff crisis, and the effort to unify dentistry to the Information Age, as discussed in RELEVANCY and COVIDCONOMICS, THE DENTAL INDUSTRY.

ALPHA LADDERS -075
CAPTAIN OF YOUR DESTINY
BY Dr. BAK NGUYEN & JONAS DIOP

In ALPHA LADDERS, Dr. Bak is sharing his private conversation and board meetings with 2 of his trusted lieutenants, strategist Jonas Diop and international Counsellor, Brenda Garcia. As both Dr. Bak and ALPHA brands are gaining in popularity and traction, it was time to get the movement to the next level. Now, it's about building a community and helping everyone willing to become ALPHAS to find their powers. Dr. Bak is a natural recruiter of ALPHAS and peers. He also spent the last 20 years plus, training and mentoring proteges. Now comes the time to empower more and more proteges to become ALPHAS. ALPHAS LADDERS is the journey of how Dr. Bak went from a product of Conformity to rise into a force of Nature, known as a kind tornado. In ALPHA LADDERS Jonas pushed Dr. Bak to retrace each of the steps of his awakening, steps that we can break down and reproduce for ourselves. The goal is to empower each willing individual to become the ultimate Captain of his or her destiny, and to do it, again and again. Welcome to the Alphas.

ALPHA LADDERS 2 -081
SHAPING LEADERS AND ACHIEVERS
BY Dr. BAK NGUYEN & BRENDA GARCIA

In ALPHA LADDERS 2, Dr. Bak is sharing the second part of his private conversation and board meetings with his trusted lieutenants. This time it is with international Counsellor, Brenda Garcia that the dialogue is taking place. In this second tome, the journey is taken to the next level. If the first tome was about the WHYs and the HOWs at an individual level, this tome is about the WHYs and the HOWs at the societal level. Through the lens of her background in international relations and diplomacy, Brenda now has the mission to help Dr. Bak establish structures, not only for his emerging organization and legacy, THE ALPHAS, but to also inspire all the other leaders and structures of our society. To do this, Brenda is taking Dr. Bak on an anthropological, sociological and philosophical journey to revisit different historical key moments in various fields and eras, going as far back as ancient Greece at the dawn of democracy, all the way to the golden era of modern multilateralism embodied by the UN structure. Learning from the legacies of prominent figures going from Plato to Ban Ki-Moon, Martin Luther King or Nelson Mandela, to Machiavelli, Marx and Simone de Beauvoir, Brenda and Dr. Bak are attempting to grasp the essence of structure and hierarchy, their goal being to empower each willing individual to become the ultimate Captain of their success, to climb up the ladders no matter how high it is, and to build their legacy one step at a time.

ALPHA MASTERMIND vol. 1 116
THE SUPERHERO'S SYNDROME
BY Dr. BAK NGUYEN

ALPHA MASTERMIND, THE SUPER HERO'S SYNDROME, is not a superhero book, but it is the tale of every leader, entrepreneur, and everyday hero facing their destiny and entourage. It uncovers how society sees our best elements and expects from them. It covers how family and friends feel and why they act as they do. But most importantly, it covers how Alphas can emerge unscathed from their growth to uncover their true powers and purpose. A veteran agent of change and difference maker, Dr. Bak is sharing his experience and secret of why and how surfing through family and society pressure without revolting and without kneeling. THE SUPERHERO'S SYNDROME is the first volume inspired by the MASTERMINDS sessions as Dr. Bak is mentoring Alpha apprentices. The superhero's syndrome came to the table as Alphas are struggling to fit in society, to keep their values and generosity while facing so much negativity all around. Welcome to the Alphas.

ALPHA MASTERMIND vol. 2 117
SUPERCHARGING MOMENTUM
BY Dr. BAK NGUYEN

ALPHA MASTERMIND, SUPERCHARGING MOMENTUM, is what is discussed on the Alphas' Round Table. Entrepreneurs, Professional Athletes, Coaches, they are all rising from their passion and momentum. To start was the first ACT. It wasn't easy but they did. Now as a FOOTBALL star, what can be next, not to fall as a HAS BEEN? You wrote your first book, what is next? What comes next after 100 books?There are so many paths to finding your powers but there is only one that I know that will keep feeding them: MOMENTUM. If discovering your powers and purposes was a great journey, the sequel to that story is a much harder one to write, to walk, to thrive from. In every story, the hero needs to rise and to grow. How can one grow even more? SUPERCHARGING MOMENTUM is the 2nd volume inspired by the MASTERMINDS sessions as Dr. Bak is mentoring Alpha apprentices. Dr. Bak is not teaching, he is sharing what he faces and does to write his next life chapter, renewing and reinventing himself again and again. Welcome to the Alphas.

ALPHA MASTERMIND vol. 3 118
RIDING DESTINY
BY Dr. BAK NGUYEN

In ALPHA MASTERMIND, RIDING DESTINY, Dr. Bak is taking you and his apprentices on the quest of rising. It will be for each to find their purpose and destiny, but the way leading there will be eased with Dr. Bak's guidance. To discover power was only the beginning, to yield power was a preparation journey, now it is about rendering power into a stream of ripple effect. "KNOW YOURSELF, KNOW THE OTHER, AND ONLY THEN, DEAL." - Dr. BAK. Well, the 2 first volumes were about knowing oneself, this one is about knowing the other and to start dealing. Once one finds power, it is barely the beginning of his or her quest. The process is not an easy one, going through separation, rejection, and denial. Then, there will be encounters of a new kind, those liberating instead of attaching.RIDING DESTINY, is the third volume inspired by the MASTERMINDS sessions as Dr. Bak is mentoring Alpha apprentices. This is about ROI on the energy invested and the one generated. Welcome to the Alphas.

AMONGST THE ALPHAS -058
BY Dr. BAK NGUYEN, with Dr. MARIA KUNSTADTER, Dr. PAUL OUELLETTE and Dr. JEREMY KRELL

In AMONGST THE ALPHAS, Dr. Bak opens the blueprint of the next level with the hope that everyone can be better, bigger, and wiser, but above all, a philosophy of Life that if, well applied, can bring inspiration to life. The Alphas rose in the midst of the COVID war as an International Collaboration to empower individuals to rise from the global crisis. Joining Dr. Bak are some of the world thinkers and achievers, the Alphas. Doctors, business people, thinkers, achievers, and influencers, are coming together to define what is an Alpha and his or her role, making the world a better place. This isn't the American dream, it is the human dream, one that can help you make History. Joining Dr. Bak are 3 Alpha authors, Dr. Maria Kunstadter, Dr. Paul Ouellette and Dr. Jeremy Krell. This book started with questions from coach Jonas Diop. Welcome to the Alphas.

AMONGST THE ALPHAS vol.2 -059
ON THE OTHER SIDE
BY Dr. BAK NGUYEN with Dr. JULIO REYNAFARJE, Dr. LINA DUSEVICIUTE and Dr. DUC-MINH LAM-DO

In AMONGST THE ALPHAS 2, Dr. Bak continues to explore the meaning of what it is to be an Alpha and how to act amongst Alphas, because as the saying taught us: alone one goes fast, together we go far. Some people see the problem. Some people look at the problem, some people created the problem. Some people leverage the problem into solutions and opportunities. Well, all of those people are Alphas. Networking and leveraging one another, their powers and reach are beyond measure. And one will keep the other in line too. Joining Dr. Bak are 3 Alphas from around the world coming together to share and collaborate, Dr. DUSEVICIUTE, Dr. LAM-DO and Dr. REYNAFARJE. This isn't the American dream, it is the human dream, one that can help you make History. Welcome to the Alphas.

AU PAYS DES PAPAS 106
BY Dr. BAK NGUYEN & WILLIAM BAK

On ne nait pas papa. On le devient. Dans sa quête d'être le meilleur papa possible pour William, Dr. Bak monte au pays des papas avec William à la recherche du papa parfait. Comme pour tout dans la vie, il doit exister une recette pour faire des papas parfaits. AU PAYS DES PAPAS est le recit des souvenirs des papas que Dr. Bak a croisé avant, alors et après qu'il soit devenu papa lui aussi. Une histoire drôle et innocente pour un Noël magique, ceci est la nouvelle aventure de William et de son papa, le Dr. Bak. Entre les livres de poulet, LEGENDS OF DESTINY et les des livres parentaux de Dr. Bak, AU PAYS DES PAPAS nous amène dans le monde magique de ces êtres magiques qui forgent des rêves, des vies et des destins.

AU PAYS DES PAPAS 2 108
BY Dr. BAK NGUYEN & WILLIAM BAK

On ne nait pas papa, ça on le sait après le premier voyage AU PAYS DES PAPAS. Suite à leur première expédition, Dr. Bak et William ont compris qu'il n'y a pas de papas parfaits ni de recette pour faire des papas parfaits. Pourtant, les papas parfaits existent! Dans ce 2e récit AU PAYS DES PAPAS, William revient avec son papa, Dr. Bak, mais cette fois, c'est William qui dirige l'expédition. Même s'il n'existe pas de recette pour faire des papas parfaits, il doit toutefois exister des façons de rendre son papa meilleur, version 2.0! C'est la nouvelle quête de William et du Dr. Bak, à la recherche de la mise-à-jour parfaite pour le meilleur papa 2.0 possible! William est déterminé à tout pour trouver la recette cette fois-ci! AU PAYS DES PAPAS 2 est le nouveau récit des aventures père-fils du Dr. Bak et de William Bak, après AU PAYS DES PAPAS 1, les livres de poulets, LEGENDS OF DESTINY et les BOOKS OF LEGENDS.

B

BOOTCAMP -071
BOOKS TO REWRITE MINDSETS INTO WINNING STATES OF MIND
BY Dr. BAK NGUYEN

In BOOTCAMP 8 BOOKS TO REWRITE MINDSETS INTO WINNING STATES OF MIND, Dr. Bak is taking you into his past, before the visionary entrepreneur, before the world records, before the Industry's disruptor status. Here are 8 of the books that changed Dr. Bak's thinking and, therefore, reset his evolution into the course we now know him for. BOOTCAMP: 8 BOOKS TO REWRITE MINDSETS INTO WINNING STATES OF MIND, is a Bootcamp of 8 weeks for anyone looking to experience Dr. Bak's training to become THE Dr. BAK you came to know and love. This book will summarize how each title changed Dr. Bak's mindset into a state of mind and how he applied that to rewrite his destiny. 8 books to read, that's 8 weeks of Bootcamp to access the power of your MIND and your WILL. Are you ready for a change?

BRANDING -044
BALANCING STRATEGY AND EMOTIONS
BY Dr. BAK NGUYEN

BRANDING is communication to its most powerful state. Branding is not just about communicating anymore but about making a promise, about establishing a relationship, and about generating an emotion. More than once, Dr. Bak proved himself to be a master, communicating and branding his ideas into flags attracting interest and influence, nationally and internationally. In BRANDING, Dr. Bak shares a very unique and personal journey, branding Dr. Bak. How does he go from Dr. Nguyen, a loved and respected dentist to becoming Dr. Bak, a world anchor hosting THE ALPHAS in the medical and financial world? More than a personal journey, BRANDING helps to break down the steps to elevate someone with nothing else but the force of his or her spirit. Welcome to the Alphas.

C

405

the parallels and the difference of both worlds, but mainly, the recipe for leveraging from one to succeed in the other, from champions and entrepreneurs to WINNERS. Build and score your millions, it is a matter of mindset! This is CHAMPION MINDSET.

COMMENT ÉCRIRE UN LIVRE EN 30 JOURS -102
PAR Dr. BAK NGUYEN

Dans COMMENT ÉCRIRE UN LIVRE EN 30 JOURS, après plus de 100 livres écrits en 4 ans, le Dr Bak revisite son premier succès, le livre dans lequel il a partagé son art et sa structure d'écriture de livres. Encore et encore, le Dr Bak a prouvé que non seulement le contenu est important, mais ce sont la structure et le processus qui rendent les livres. L'inspiration n'est que le début. Si vous envisagez d'écrire votre premier livre, ceci est votre chance. Si vous y pensez, faites-le, et aussi vite que possible. Écrire votre premier livre vous libérera de votre passé et vous ouvrira les portes de votre avenir! Tout le monde a une histoire qui mérite d'être partagée! Par où commencer, comment passer le MUR DE L'INSPIRATION, quelles sont les techniques pour apporter de la profondeur à votre histoire, comment structurer votre chapitre, combien de chapitres, comment avoir un livre, en un mois? Voilà les réponses que vous trouverez dans COMMENT ÉCRIRE UN LIVRE EN 30 JOURS. Vous trouverez un trésor de sagesse, un mentor et surtout, une confiance renouvelée pour écrire, que ce soit, votre premier, deuxième ou même 10e livre. Au fait, le Dr. Bak a écrit ce livre et l'a fait publier en 6 jours. Bienvenu(e)s aux Alphas.

COMMENT ÉCRIRE 2 LIVRES EN 10 JOURS -115
Par WILLIAM & Dr. BAK NGUYEN

Dans COMMENT ÉCRIRE 2 LIVRES EN 10 JOURS, William Bak s'attaque au succès de son père, COMMENT ÉCRIRE UN LIVRE EN 30 JOURS. Cette fois-ci, père et fils font équipe pour vous partager l'art d'écrire de la fiction. Comme le titre le mentionne, William doit écrire ce livre et le suivant en 10 jours. Pour ne pas vous induire en erreur, écrire votre premier livre de fiction prendra plus que 10 jours. Cependant, les procédés contenus dans ce livre vous aideront à accélérer votre production et à porter votre créativité à des niveaux inégalés. William a 12 ans et déjà, il a signé 36 livres dont la plupart sont de la fiction. En ce sens, il est un vétéran auteur, un qui a connu les hauts et les bas du manque d'inspiration. Au côté de William, Dr. Bak se prête aussi au jeux de démolir son propre succès et le remplacer par une nouvelle marque. Père et fils, ils vous partagent leurs secrets et expérience à écrire un duo-choque depuis les derniers 4 ans. COMMENT ÉCRIRE 2 LIVRES EN 10 JOURS a commencé par une farce qui est rapidement devenu leur plus grand défi à ce jour, d'écrire 2 livres en 10 jours. Bienvenu(e)s aux Alphas.

COVIDCONOMIE - 111
CONTRER L'INFLATION SANS TOUCHER LES TAUX D'INTÉRÊT
PAR Dr. BAK NGUYEN, ANDRÉ CHÂTEALAIN, TRANIE VO, FRANÇOIS DUFOUR, WILLIAM BAK

COVIDCONOMIE est l'ensemble des observations, analyses des phénomènes démographiques et économiques secondaires à la pandémie de la COVID-19. CONTRER L'INFLATION SANS TOUCHER LES TAUX D'INTÉRÊT, est la réflexion et plan macro des ALPHAS pour le CANADA et les ETATS-UNIS D'AMÉRIQUE dans un premier temps et un modèle économique pour l'ensemble des pays d'Occident.Joint par des leaders en finance et en économie, dont André Châtelain, ancien premier vice-président du MOUVEMENT DESJARDINS, le Dr. Bak met la table à des discussions inclusives et constructives pouvant changer le cours de l'Histoire dans l'intérêt des citoyens au quotidien.CONTRER L'INFLATION SANS TOUCHER LES TAUX D'INTÉRÊT, est un mémoire collectif des ALPHAS pour lutter contre l'inflation post-pandémique et éviter une récession internationale globale.

COVIDCONOMICS - 112
TAMING INFLATION WITHOUT INCREASING INTEREST RATES
BY Dr. BAK NGUYEN, ANDRÉ CHÂTEALAIN, TRANIE VO, FRANÇOIS DUFOUR, WILLIAM BAK

COVIDCONOMICS, are the reflections, analysis and discussion of the ALPHAS, hosted by Dr. Bak to understand the demographic et economical trends post-COVID 19. TAMING INFLATION WITHOUT INCREASING INTEREST RATES is a macro plan by the ALPHAS for Canada and the USA which can inspire a new economical model for all of the Western worlds. Joined by leaders in finance as André Châtelain, former 1st Vice-President of the MOUVEMENT DESJARDINS, Dr. Bak is hosting an inclusive discussion to save our economy in these very troubled times as the country is still looking to get back on its feet from the Pandemic while wars are raging on multiple fronts. TAMING INFLATION WITHOUT INCREASING INTEREST RATES is our proposal to save the economy and our recovery from a global recession.

E

EMPOWERMENT -069
BY Dr. BAK NGUYEN

In EMPOWERMENT, Dr. Bak's 69th book, writing a book every 8 days for 8 weeks in a row to write the next world record of writing 72 books/36 months, Dr. Bak is taking a rest, sharing his inner feelings, inspiration, and motivation. Much more than his dairy, EMPOWERMENT is the key to walking in his footsteps and comprehending the process of an overachiever. Dr. Bak's helped and inspired countless people to find their voice, to live their dream, and to be the better version of themselves. Why is he sharing as much and keep sharing? Why is he going that fast, always further and further, why and how is he keeping his inspiration and momentum? Those are all the answers EMPOWERMENT will deliver to you. This book might be one of the fastest Dr. Bak has written, not because of time constraints but from inspiration, pure inspiration to share and to grow. There is always a dark side to each power, two faces to a coin. Well, this is the less prominent facet of Dr. Bak's Momentum and success, the road to his MINDSET.

F

FORCES OF NATURE 015
FORGING THE CHARACTER OF WINNERS

BY Dr. BAK NGUYEN

In FORCES OF NATURE, Dr. Bak is giving his all. This is his 15 books written within 15 months. It is the end of a marathon to set the next world record. For the occasion, he wanted to end with a big bang! How about a book with all of his biggest challenges? In a Quest of Identity, a journey looking for his name and powers, Dr. Bak is borrowing myths and legends to make this journey universal. Yes, this is Dr. Bak's mythology. Demons, heroes and Gods, there are forces of Nature that we all meet on our way for our name. Some will scare us, some will fight us, and some will manipulate us. We can flee, we can hide, we can fight. What we do will define our next encounter and the one after. A tale of personal growth, a journey to find power and purpose, Dr. Bak is showing us the path to freedom, the Path of Life. Welcome to the Alphas.

H

HORIZON, BUILDING UP THE VISION -045
VOLUME ONE
BY Dr. BAK NGUYEN

Dr. Bak is opening up to your demand! Many of you are following Dr. Bak online and are asking to know more about his lifestyle. This is how he has chosen to respond: sharing his lifestyle as he travelled the world and what he learnt in each city to come to build his Mindset as a driver and a winner. Here are 10 destinations (over 69 that will be followed in the next volumes...) in which he shares his journey. New York, Quebec, Paris, Punta Cana, Monaco, Los Angeles, Nice, and Holguin, the journey happened over twenty years.

HORIZON, ON THE FOOTSTEP OF TITANS -048
VOLUME TWO
BY Dr. BAK NGUYEN

Dr. Bak is opening up to your demand! Many of you are following Dr. Bak online and are asking to know more about his lifestyle. This is how he has chosen to respond: sharing his lifestyle as he travelled the world and what he learnt in each city to come to build his Mindset as a driver and a winner. Here are 9 destinations (over 72 that will follow in the next volumes...) in which he shares his journey. Hong Kong, London, Rome, San Francisco, Anaheim, and more..., the journey happened over twenty years. Dr. Bak is sharing with you his feelings, impressions, and how they shaped his state of mind and character into Dr. Bak. From a dreamer to a driver and a builder, the journey started when he was 3. Wealth is a state of mind, and a state of mind is the basis of the drive. Find out about the mind of an Industry's disruptor.

HOW TO WRITE A BOOK IN 30 DAYS -042
BY Dr. BAK NGUYEN

In HOW TO WRITE A BOOK IN 30 DAYS, after more than 100 books written in 4 years, Dr. Bak is revisiting his first hit, the book in which he shared his craft and structure of how to write books. After 100 books, Dr. Bak proved that not only content is important, but what will keep the words coming are the structure and the process. If you are looking into writing your first book, this is your chance. If you are thinking about it, do it, and as fast as possible. Writing your first book will set you free from your past and open the doors to your own future! Everyone has a story worth telling! Where to start, how to get by the INSPIRATIONAL WALL, what are the techniques to bring depth into your storytelling, how to structure your chapter, how many chapters, how to have a book, in a month? These are the answers you will find within HOW TO WRITE A BOOK IN 30 DAYS. You will find a wealth of wisdom from his experience writing your first, second or even 10th book. Dr. Bak is sharing his secrets writing books. By the way, he wrote this book and got it published within 6 days. Welcome to the Alphas.

HOW 2 WRITE 2 BOOKS IN 10 DAYS -114
BY WILLIAM & Dr. BAK NGUYEN

HOW 2 WRITE 2 BOOKS IN 10 DAYS, is William Bak takes on his father's hit, HOW TO WRITE A BOOK IN 30 DAYS. This time, William is covering the art of writing fiction. As mentioned in the title, William is writing this book and the next one within 10 days. Just not to mislead you, writing fiction will take longer, but once you have done all your prep work and research, it can be written as quickly. William is only 12 and already, he has signed 35 books. Most of his books are fiction, so on the matter, he is a veteran author, one with much experience of the ups and downs when it comes to writing books and getting them to the finish line Joining him is Dr. Bak who is sharing his secrets of writing fiction too. What does it take, how different it is from writing non-fictional books and what does it take to inspire and motivate his 12-year-old son to write as much, matching his world record pace? HOW 2 WRITE 2 BOOKS IN 10 DAYS is a joke between 2 world record authors teasing one another as they keep raising the bar higher and higher. Welcome to the Alphas.

HOW TO WRITE A SUCCESSFUL BUSINESS PLAN -049
BY Dr. BAK NGUYEN & ROUBA SAKR

In HOW TO WRITE A SUCCESSFUL BUSINESS PLAN, Dr. Bak is given 20 plus years of experience and knowledge of what it is to be an entrepreneur and more importantly, how to have the investors and banks on your side. Being an entrepreneur is surely not something you learn from school, but there are steps to master so you can communicate your views and vision. That's the only way you will have financing. Writing a business is only not a mandatory stop only for the bankers, but an essential step for every entrepreneur, to know the direction and what's coming next. A business plan is also not set in stone, if there is a truth in business is that nothing will go as planned. Writing down your business plan the first time will prepare you to adapt and overcome the challenges and surprises. For most entrepreneurs, a business is a passion. To most investors and all banks, a business is a system. Your business plan is the map to that system. However unique your ideas and business are, the mapping follows the same steps and pattern.

HOW TO SEDUCE ANYONE 129
BY Dr. BAK NGUYEN

In HOW TO SEDUCE ANYONE, Dr. Bak is pushed by 2 of his female apprentices to share the secret behind his smile and influence. Seduction has many facets and can be leveraged in so many ways. Dr. Bak's way is to seduce without seducing, with tricks or fireworks. He, himself never saw himself as a seducer, until asked to share his skills and knowledge on the matter. Everything in life is about connecting and interacting with others. So it is safe to say that all of our social life is about seducing, even when sharing. To learn to eat, to talk, to wrap, and to open is an old Vietnamese saying about the ways of life. Well, to Dr. Bak, it is much simpler than that. Seduction is about being confident enough to be available to the other person, available to listen and to empower. It is all about what the other person feels in your presence which is the key to your influence and charm. Easier said than done! Well in this journey, you are following Dr. Bak along with Alpha Coach Mel and Alpha host Natasha DG to uncover the ways to seduce without seducing, to gain the minds and hearts of those you touch without compromising or overselling yourself. HOW TO SEDUCE ANYONE is a conversation with Dr. Bak, straight from the heart and without filtre. Based on a podcast interview from WOMAN UP and more than 3 decades of winning the hearts of those he touches, these are Dr. Bak's secrets. Welcome to the Alphas.

HUMILITY FOR SUCCESS 051
BALANCING STRATEGY AND EMOTIONS
BY Dr. BAK NGUYEN

HUMILITY FOR SUCCESS is exploring the emotional discomforts and challenges champions, and overachievers put themselves through. Success is never done overnight and on the way, just like the pain and the struggles aren't enough, we are dealing with the doubts, the haters, and those who like to tell us how to live our lives and what to do. At the same time, nothing of worth can be achieved alone. Every legend has a cast of characters, allies, mentors, companions, rivals, and foes. So one needs the key to social behaviour. HUMILITY FOR SUCCESS is exploring the matter and will help you sort out beliefs from values, and peers from friends. Humility is much more about how we see ourselves than how others see us. For any entrepreneur and champion, our daily is to set our mindset right, and to perfect our skills, not to fit in. There is a world where CONFIDENCE grows in synergy with HUMILITY. As you set the right label on the right belief, you will be able to grow and leave the lies and haters far behind. This is HUMILITY FOR SUCCESS.

HYBRID -011
THE MODERN QUEST OF IDENTITY
BY Dr. BAK NGUYEN

I

IDENTITY -004
THE ANTHOLOGY OF QUESTS
BY Dr. BAK NGUYEN

What if John Lennon was still alive and running for president today? What kind of campaign will he be running? IDENTIFY -THE ANTHOLOGY OF QUESTS is about the quest each of us has to undertake, sooner or later, THE QUEST OF IDENTITY. Citizens of the world, aim to be one, the one, one whole, one unity, made of many. That's the anthology of life! Start with your one, find your unity, and your legend will start. We are all small-minded people anyway! We need each other to be one! We need each other to be happy, so we, so you, so I, can be happy. This is the chorus of life. This is our song! Citizens of the world, I salute you! This is the first tome of the IDENTITY QUEST. FORCES OF NATURE (tome 2) will be following in SUMMER 2021. Also under development, Tome 3 - THE CONQUEROR WITHIN will start production soon.

INDUSTRIES DISRUPTORS -006
BY Dr. BAK NGUYEN

INDUSTRIES DISRUPTORS   is a strange title, one that sparkles mixed feelings. A disruptor is someone making a difference, and since we, in general, do not like change, the label is mostly negative. But a disruptor is mostly someone who sees the same problem and challenge from another angle. The disruptor will tackle that angle and come up with something new from something existent. That's evolution! In INDUSTRIES DISRUPTORS, Dr. Bak is joining forces with James Stephan-Usypchuk to share with us what is going on in the minds and shoes of those entrepreneurs disrupting the old habits. Dr. Bak is changing the world from a dental chair, disrupting the dental, and now the book industry. James is a maverick in the Intelligence space, from marketing to Artificial Intelligence. Coming from very different backgrounds and industries, they end up telling very similar stories. If disruptors change the world, well, their story proves that disruptors can be made and forged. Here's the recipe. Here are their stories.

K

KRYPTO -040
TO SAVE THE WORLD
BY Dr. BAK NGUYEN & ILYAS BAKOUCH

L

L'ART DE TRANSFORMER DE LA SOUPE EN MAGIE -103
PAR Dr. BAK NGUYEN

Dans L'ART DE TRANSFORMER DE LA SOUPE EN MAGIE, Dr. Bak remonte aux sources pour connaître la source de son génie et la recette qui a été transféré à son fils, William Bak, auteur et record mondial dès l'âge de 8 ans. Docteur en médecine dentaire, entrepreneur, écrivain record mondial, musicien, Dr. Bak est d'abord et avant tout un fils qui a une maman qui croit en lui. L'ART DE TRANSFORMER DE LA SOUPE EN MAGIE est dédié à la recette du génie, celle qui pousse une mère a mijoté les ingrédients de l'espoir dans un bouillon d'amour, à y ajuster un zeste de bonheur et un brin d'ambition. Dans la lignée des livres parentaux de Dr. Bak, L'ART DE TRANSFORMER DE LA SOUPE EN MAGIE est dédié à la première femme dans sa vie, celle qui a tracé son destin et celle qui l'a cultivée.

LEADERSHIP -003
PANDORA'S BOX
BY Dr. BAK NGUYEN

LEADERSHIP, PANDORA'S BOX is 21 presidential speeches for a better tomorrow for all of us. It aims to drive HOPE and motivation into each and every one of us. Together we can make the difference, we hold such power. Covering themes from LOYALTY to GENEROSITY, from FREEDOM and INTELLIGENCE to DOUBTS and DEATH, this is not the typical presidential or motivational speeches that we are used to. LEADERSHIP PANDORA'S BOX will surf your emotions first, only to dive with you to touch the core and soul of our meaning: to matter. This is not a Quest of Identity, but the cry to rally as a species, raise our heads toward the future and move forward as a WHOLE. Not a typical Dr. Bak's book, LEADERSHIP, PANDORA'S BOX is a must-read for all of you looking for hope and purpose, all of us, citizens of the world.

LEADERSHIP vol. 1 (ALPHA DENTISTRY) -121
CHANGING THE WORLD FROM A DENTAL CHAIR

ALBANIA BRAZIL CANADA HUNGARY MALAYSIA SPAIN USA

BY Dr. BAK NGUYEN, Dr. MAHSA KHAGHANI, Dr. NAGY KATALIN, with guest authors Dr. PAUL DOMINIQUE, Dr. PAUL OUELLETTE, Dr. GURIEN DEMIRAQI, Dr. BENNETE FERNANDES, Dr. SANDRA FABIANO, Dr. ARASH HAKHAMIAN and Dr. MARILYN SANDOR

ALPHA DENTISTRY proudly presents LEADERSHIP, CHANGING THE WORLD FROM A DENTAL CHAIR. This time, Dr. Bak is leading the charge of rebuilding the foundations of the dental industry, especially after the light shed by COVID. More than once, populations from all around the world have expressed their negative perceptions and uneasy feelings about the dental industry. For decades, we turned deaf and blinded to these criticisms. In the worse health crisis of our lifetime, our specialists, experts and all our doctors were benched, despite being health professionals... The message is clear, the whole field must be rethought and better adapted to our modern societies. In the hope of bringing new ideas and philosophies, Dr. Bak is joined by Dr. Mahsa Khaghani from Spain and Dr. Nagy Katalin from Hungary, along with Dr. Paul Dominique, Dr. Paul Ouellette, Dr. Arash Hakhamian and Dr. Marilyn Sandor from the USA, Dr. Gurien Demiraqi from Albania, Dr. Bennete Fernandes from Malaysia, and Dr. Sandra Fabiano from Brazil to lead this history journey looking to modernize and make dentistry more accessible and affordable. It will take leadership and courage to assemble all of the world's dental industry and bridge the gaps to a better future. It starts by listening and then, dialoguing. LEADERSHIP is an inclusive dialogue. This is the first volume of this new series in which International Dental leaders will be joining forces to rebuild Dentistry. First mission: lower the costs of dentistry. Welcome to the Alphas.

LEGENDS OF DESTINY vol.1 -101
THE PROLOGUES OF DESTINY
BY Dr. BAK NGUYEN & WILLIAM BAK

The war between the forces of death and the legions of life lasted for centuries, ravaging most of the twin planets, Destiny and Earth. The end was so imminent that even the Gods got involved to save Life from eternal doom. Heroes rise and fall from all sides. Some fight for good, others, for evil. Gods, titans, angels, and demons all took sides in the war. Gods fight and kill other gods. Angel fights alongside demons, striking down Gods and Titans, and rival angels. The war lasted for so long that no one even remembers what they were fighting for. Some fight for domination while others, just to survive. The war ravages Destiny, the twin sister of planet Earth to the brink of annihilation. All eyes now turn to Earth. As the balance of the creation itself hands in the balance, a species emerges as holding the balance to victory: mankind. For the future of Humanity, of Gods and men and everything in between, this is the last stand of Destiny, a last chance for life.

LEGENDS OF DESTINY vol.2 -107
THE BOOK OF ELVES
BY Dr. BAK NGUYEN & WILLIAM BAK

Caught between the Orcs invading from the center of Destiny, the Angels raining down and the Demons eating from within, the Elves are turning from their old beliefs and Gods for salvation. For Millennials, Elves turned to Odin and the Forces of Nature for answers and guidance. Since the imminent destruction of their kingdoms and cities, a new God is offering Hope, Kal, the old God of fire. Kal gave them more than Hope, he gave the elves who turned to him for passage to a new world. But more than hope, more than fear, Elves value honour and Destiny. At least their old guards and heroes do. With their world crumbling down, and the rise of the new and younger generations, Elf's society seems to be at the crossroad of evolution. It is convert or die. Or die fighting or die kneeling. The Book of Elves is the story of a civilization facing its fate in the blink of destruction.

LEGENDS OF DESTINY vol.3 -135
WHISPER OF DARKNESS
BY Dr. BAK NGUYEN & WILLIAM BAK

WHISPER OF DARKNESS is the 3rd volume of LEGENDS OF DESTINY. This time, the story is set at the celestial level, as the war between the angels is raging. After Adrian's ascension to power, the dissident angels left. Some stay isolated as Archangel Anton and Lucifer and will be known as the Errants.   Others will regroup and organize. Heaven calls them the Dark Angels, those no more within the light of Heaven. Between the raids to put down the Gods out of control, Heaven is also sending squadrons of Angels to hunt down the dissidents with more or less success. This is the story of angels Ethel and Eto, as they are sent on a recognition mission to uncover the whereabouts of Kohël, a dissident angel, now known as Dali, the God of the Wind. Both junior angels looking to prove their worth to Heaven, the Council of Angels, and their Angel Lord, Adrian. Well, they are not the only ones looking to make their mark, as Hasdielle, a Dark Angel, is also looking to prove Heaven weak and wrong! Follow the legend of Ethel and Eto in WHISPER OF DARKNESS, the 3rd volume of LEGENDS OF DESTINY.

LEGENDS OF DESTINY vol.4 -137
04
BY Dr. BAK NGUYEN & WILLIAM BAK

In a world where the realms of angels and gods collide, the heavens are in chaos and the fate of the universe hanging in the balance, meet Mikael, Lucifer, Xaphan, and Morieshal, angel cadets of TEAM OMEGA 4. No, their mission is not to save the universe, just to try not to break it! TEAM OMEGA 4, the cadet squadron to which ex-archangels Mikael and Lucifer are now assigned, after being demoted from Archangels to cadets. This is a legend before Adrian, the Angel Lord, it was the time when the angels were a young society, policing Creation as they were meant to do. In a time of democracy and acceptance, the angels were trying to find balance and their place in the universe. Follow cadets Lucifer and Mikael, destined to become amongst the strongest of angelkind as well as their partners in crime, angels Xaphan and Morieshal destined to become legends. This is the tale of their youth and innocence. LEGENDS OF DESTINY volume 4 - O4 is taking place before the events of Prologue of Destiny, The Book of Elves, and Whisper of Destiny. This is LEGENDS OF DESTINY.

LEGENDS OF DESTINY vol.5 138
SCROLL OF DESTINY
BY Dr. BAK NGUYEN & WILLIAM BAK

SCROLL OF THE DESTINY is the 5th volume of LEGENDS OF DESTINY. The events of this book happen between the events of O4 between episodes 2 and 3, as Mikael and Lucifer are cadets, alongside Xaphan and Morieshal as the infamous members of the Omega Squadron. As they returned from their successful mission, rescuing Sekhmet, daughter of Ra, they are sent almost immediately to the Orient, looking for mystery creatures called dragons. The orders came from the top, from Anthem herself. So this is the journey of Mikael, Lucifer, Xaphan, and Morieshal still hyped from their diplomatic success, not killing anyone. Scroll of Destiny is the new chapter in Angel annals, the kind changing the course of evolution itself. Follow the legend of young Mikael, Lucifer, Xaphan, and Morieshal as the OMEGA 4 Squadron, in SCROLL OF DESTINY, the 5th volume of LEGENDS OF DESTINY.

LEGENDS OF DESTINY tome 1 134
THE BOOK OF ANGELS
BY Dr. BAK NGUYEN & WILLIAM BAK

LEGENDS OF DESTINY, THE BOOK OF ANGELS is the Annals of the Angels of the Legends of Destiny. This book is the origin story and the fate of each of the angels and archangels from this epic fresque. As the worlds are clashing and the Gods are out of control, Ethem, the primal force created the angels to balance the forces of the universe. These are the stories of the guardians of balance, the wings of justice, and the tragedies of power and its corruption. Follow Angel Lord Adrian, Archangel Mikael, Hermes, and Lucifer from their fights to their rise and demise. Follow the adventure of Angels Eto, Ethel, Jardoo; follow the rise of Dark Angels Anak, Felice, or Hesdielle. Choose your faction, Archangel, Angels, Dark Angels, Guild, Phantoms, bionics, or hybrid, you will each time be amazed. Caught between the Gods, the Titans, the demons, the elves, the orcs, the humans, and everything in between, the Angels bear the heavy responsibility of balancing life and creation. These are their legends.

LEGENDS OF DESTINY tome 2 -136
GREEK MYTHOLOGY
BY Dr. BAK NGUYEN & WILLIAM BAK

LEGENDS OF DESTINY, GREEK MYTHOLOGY is the Annals of the Greek Gods, Heroes, monsters and mythological creatures of ancient Greek, from the Amazonians to the Atlantians, from the Olympians to the Greeks, this is our review of ancient Greece. The heroes and Gods of Greek Mythology are now available and AI ready to merge with the world of LEGENDS OF DESTINY. Follow Zeus, Poseidon, Hades, Hera, Hermes, Athena, Demeter, Artemis, Apollo, Aphrodite, Hephaestus, Ares, Dionysos, and Hestia from the heights of Mount Olympus to the depths of the sea and the depth of the Underworld. Follow the adventures of Heracles, Theseus, Achilles, Perseus, Cassandra, and so many more as you are walking in their steps, in ancient Greece. This is history, it is culture, it is drama and now, it can be yours to remake within the universe of Legends of Destiny.

LE POUVOIR DE LA SÉDUCTION -130
PAR Dr. BAK NGUYEN

Dans LE POUVOIR DE LA SÉDUCTION, le Dr Bak est poussé par deux de ses protégées Alphas à partager le secret derrière son sourire et son influence. La séduction a de nombreuses facettes et peut être utilisée à de nombreuses fins. Séduire sans séduire, est la philosophie du Dr. Bak, sans astuces ni feux d'artifice. Lui-même ne s'est jamais considéré comme un séducteur jusqu'à ce qu'on le sollicite pour ses compétences et secrets en la matière. La vie sociale est une grande séduction. Que ce soit d'interagir, partager, soigner, enseigner, même aider, tout revient sur l'aptitude de chacun à mettre en confiance. Apprendre à manger, à parler, à emballer et à ouvrir est un vieux dicton vietnamien sur la façon de vivre. Eh bien, pour le Dr Bak, c'est beaucoup plus simple que cela. La séduction consiste à être suffisamment confiant pour pouvoir s'oublier et être disponible pour l'autre. La clé de la séduction et de l'influence est dans comment les autres se sentent en notre présence. LE POUVOIR DE LA SÉDUCTION est une conversation entre avec la coach Mel et l'animatrice Natasha DG, le Dr Bak et vous. Ce livre est inspiré du podcast WOMAN UP et sur plus de 3 décennies à conquérir les cœurs et le respect de ceux qu'il touche. Voici les secrets du Dr Bak. Bienvenu(e) aux Alphas.

LEVERAGE -014
COMMUNICATION INTO SUCCESS
BY Dr. BAK NGUYEN

In LEVERAGE COMMUNICATION TO SUCCESS, Dr. Bak shares his secret and mindsets to elevate an idea into a vision and a vision into an endeavour. Some endeavours will be a project, some others will become companies, and some will grow into a movement. It does not matter, each started with great communication. Communication is a very vast concept, education, sale, sharing, empowering, coaching, preaching, and entertaining. Those are all different kinds of communication. The intent differs, the audiences vary, and the messages are unique but the frame can be templated and mastered. In LEVERAGE COMMUNICATION TO SUCCESS, Dr. Bak is loyal to his core, sharing only what he knows best, what he has done himself. This book is dedicated to communicating successfully in business.

M

MASTERMIND, 7 WAYS INTO THE BIG LEAGUE -052
BY Dr. BAK NGUYEN & JONAS DIOP

MASTERMIND, 7 WAYS INTO THE BIG LEAGUE is the result of the encounter between business coach Jonas Diop and Dr. Bak. As a professional podcaster and someone always seeking the truth and ways to leverage success and performance, coach Jonas is putting Dr. Bak to the test, one that should reveal his secret to overachieve month after month, accumulating a new world record every month. Follow those two great minds as they push each other to surpass themselves, each in their own way and own style. MASTERMIND, 7 WAYS INTO THE BIG LEAGUE is more than a roadmap to success, it is a journey and a live testimony as you are turning the pages, one by one.

MENTORSHIP -133
BY Dr. BAK NGUYEN & COACH MEL

MENTORSHIP, THE POWER OF SHARING is the conversation between a mentor and his apprentice. This is a journey of discovery, of healing, and of empowerment. Power and wisdom don't fade with time, they morph stronger and shapeless if one can renew purpose. Walking legends, writing history, even for seduction, one needs to understand and master the POWER OF MIRRORS to grow, to win. The power of mirrors is the only power that won't corrupt its host. It might blind, but not corrupt. And the only way to avoid blindness in the light of great power is to have a mirror to react to. This is the essence of a mentor/apprentice relationship. To the apprentice, it is the privilege to gain much power and wisdom. To the mentor, it is the chance to break the limits of his or her own power to ascend into even greater power. MENTORSHIP, THE POWER OF SHARING is the conversation between Dr. Bak and Coach Mel, on her path to setting the next world record mark in literature, beating her mentor. It is the universal dynamic of every mentor-apprentice synergy. Welcome to the Alphas.

MIDAS TOUCH -065
POST-COVID DENTISTRY
BY Dr. BAK NGUYEN, Dr. JULIO REYNAFARJE AND Dr. PAUL OUELLETTE

MIDAS TOUCH, is the memoir of what happened in the ALPHAS SUMMIT in the midst of the GREAT PAUSE as great minds throughout the world in the dental field are coming together. As the time of competition is obsolete, the new era of collaboration is blooming. This is the 3rd book of the ALPHAS, after AFTERMATH and RELEVANCY, all written in the midst of confinement. Dr. Julio Reynafarje is bearing this initiative, to share with you the secret of a successful and lasting relationship with your patients, balancing science and psychology, kindness, and professionalism. He personally invited the ALPHAS to join as co-author, Dr. Paul Ouellette, Dr. Paul Dominique, and Dr. Bak. Together, they have more than 100 years of combined experience, wisdom, trade, skills, philosophy, and secrets to share with you to empower you in the rebuilding of the dental profession in the aftermath of COVID. RELEVANCY was about coming together and rebuilding the future. MIDAS TOUCH is about how to build, one treatment plan at a time, one story at a time, one smile at a time.

MINDSET ARMORY -050
BY Dr. BAK NGUYEN

MINDSET ARMORY is Dr. Bak's 49th book, days after he completed his world record of writing 48 books within 24 months, on top of being the CEO of Mdex & Co and a full-time cosmetic dentist. Dr. Bak is undoubtedly an OVERACHIEVER. In his last books, he has shared more and more of his lifestyle and how it forged his winning mindset. Within MINDSET ARMORY, Dr. Bak is sharing with us his tools, how he found them, forged them, and leverage them. Just like any warrior needs a shield, a sword, and a ride, here are Dr. Bak's. For any entrepreneur, the road to success is a long and winding journey. On the way, some will find allies and foes. Some allies will become foes, and some foes might become allies. In today's competitive world, the only constant is change. With the right tool, it is possible to achieve. The right tool, the right mindset. This is MINDSET ARMORY.

MIRROR-085
BY Dr. BAK NGUYEN

MIRROR is the theme for a personal book. Not only to Dr. Bak but to all of us looking to reach beyond who and what we actually are. MIRROR is special in the fact that it is not only the content of the book that is of worth but the process in which Dr. Bak shared his own evolution. To go beyond who we are, one must grow every day. And how do you compare your growth and how far have you reached? Looking in the mirror. In all of Dr. Bak's writing, looking at the past is a trap to avoid at all costs. Looking in the mirror, is that any better? Share Dr. Bak's way to push and keep pushing himself without friction or resistance. Please read that again. To evolve without friction or resistance... that is the source of infinite growth and the unification of the Quest for Power and the Quest of Happiness.

MOMENTUM TRANSFER 009
BY Dr. BAK NGUYEN & Coach DINO MASSON

How to be successful in your business and life? Achieve Your Biggest Goals With MOMENTUM TRANSFER. START THE BUSINESS YOU WANT - AND BRING IT NEXT LEVEL! GET THE LIFE YOU ALWAYS WANTED - AND IMPROVE IT! TAKE ANY PROJECTS YOU HAVE - AND MAKE THEM THE BEST! In this powerful book, you'll discover what a small business owner learnt from a millionaire and successful entrepreneur. He applied his mentor's principles and is explaining them in full detail in this book. The small business owner wrote the book he has always wanted to read and went from the verge of bankruptcy to quadrupling his revenues in less than 9 months and improve his personal life by increasing his energy and bringing back peacefulness. Together, the millionaire and the small business owner are sharing their most valuable business and life lessons with the world. The most powerful book to increase your momentum in your business and your life introduces simple and radical life-changing concepts: Multiply your business revenues by finding the Eye of your Momentum - Increase your energy by building and feeding your own Momentum - How to increase your confidence with these simple steps - How to transfer your new powerful energy into other aspects of your business and life - How to set goals and achieve them (even crush them!)- How to always tap into an effortless and limitless force within you- And much, much more!

P

PLAYBOOK INTRODUCTION -055
BY Dr. BAK NGUYEN

In PLAYBOOK INTRODUCTION, Dr. Bak is open the door to all the newcomers and aspirant entrepreneurs who are looking at where and when to start. Based on questions of two college students wanting to know how to start their entrepreneurial journey, Dr. Bak dives into his experiences to empower the next generation, not about what they should do, but how he, Dr. Bak, would have done it today. This is an important aspect to recognize in the business world, the world has changed since the INFORMATION AGE and the advent of the millenniums into the market. Most matrix and know-how have to be adapted to today's speed and accessibility to the information. We are living at the INFORMATION AGE, this book is the precursor to the ABUNDANCE AGE, at least to those open to embracing the opportunity.

PLAYBOOK INTRODUCTION 2 -056
BY Dr. BAK NGUYEN

In PLAYBOOK INTRODUCTION 2, Dr. Bak continues the journey to welcome the newcomers and aspirant entrepreneurs looking at where and when to start. If the first volume covers the mindset, the second is covering much more in-depth the concept of debt and leverage. This is an important aspect to recognize in the business world, the world has changed since the INFORMATION AGE and the advent of the millenniums into the market. Most matrix and know-how have to be adapted to today's speed and accessibility to the information. We are living at the INFORMATION AGE, this book is the precursor to the ABUNDANCE AGE, at least to those open to embrace the opportunity.

POWER -043
EMOTIONAL INTELLIGENCE
BY Dr. BAK NGUYEN

IN POWER, EMOTIONAL INTELLIGENCE, Dr. Bak is sharing his experiences and secrets leveraging on his EMOTIONAL INTELLIGENCE, a power we all have within. From SYMPATHY, having others opening up to you, to ACTIVE LISTENING, saving you time and energy; from EMPATHY, allowing you to predict the future to INFLUENCE, enabling you to draft the future, not to forget the power of the crowd with MOMENTUM, you are now in possession of power in tune with nature, yourself. It is a unique take on the subject to empower you to find your powers and your destiny. Visionary businessman, and doctor in dentistry, Dr. Bak describes himself as a Dentist by circumstances, a communicator by passion, and an entrepreneur by nature.

POWERPLAY 078
HOW TO BUILD THE PERFECT TEAM
BY Dr. BAK NGUYEN

In POWERPLAY, HOW TO BUILD THE PERFECT TEAM, Dr. Bak is sharing with you his experience, perspective, and mistake travelling the journey of the entrepreneur. A serial entrepreneur himself, he started venture only with a single partner as a team to build companies with a director of human resources and a board of directors. POWERPLAY is not a story, it is the HOW TO build the perfect team, knowing that perfection is a lie. So how can one build a team that will empower his or her vision? How to recruit, how to train, how to retain? Those are all legitimate questions. And all of those won't matter if the first question isn't answered: what is the reason for the team? There is the old way to hire and the new way to recruit. Yes, Human Resources is all about mindset too! This journey is one of introspection. of leadership, and a cheat sheet to build, not only the perfect team but the team that will empower your legacy to the next level.

PROFESSION HEALTH - TOME ONE 005
THE UNCONVENTIONAL QUEST OF HAPPINESS
BY Dr. BAK NGUYEN, Dr. MIRJANA SINDOLIC, Dr. ROBERT DURAND AND COLLABORATORS

Why are health professionals burning out while they give the best of themselves to heal the world? Dr. Bak aims to break the curse of isolation that health professionals face and establish a conversation to start the healing process. PROFESSION HEALTH is the basis of an ongoing discussion and will also serve as an introduction to a study led by Professor Robert Durand, DMD, MSc Science from the University of Montreal, a study co-financed by Mdex and the Federal Government of Canada. Co-writers are Dr. Mirjana Sindolic, Professor Robert Durand, Dr. Jean De Serres, MD and former President of Hema Quebec, Counsel-Minister Luis Maria Kalaff Sanchez, Dr. Miguel Angel Russo, MD, Banker Anthony Siggia, Banker Kyles Yves, and more… This is the first Tome of three, dedicated to helping "WHITE COATS" to heal and to find their happiness.

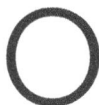

O

04-136
LEGENDS OF DESTINY VOL. 4
BY Dr. BAK NGUYEN & WILLIAM BAK

In a world where the realms of angels and gods collide, the heavens are in chaos and the fate of the universe hanging in the balance, meet Mikael, Lucifer, Xaphan, and Morieshal, angel cadets of TEAM OMEGA 4. No, their mission in not to save the universe, just to try not to break it! TEAM OMEGA 4, the cadet squadron to which ex-archangels Mikael and Lucifer are now assigned, after being demoted from Archangels to cadets. This is a legend before Adrian, the Angel Lord, it was the time when the angels were a young society, policing Creation as they were meant to do. In a time of democracy and acceptance, the angels were trying to find balance and their place in the universe. Follow cadets Lucifer and Mikael, destined to become amongst the strongest of angelkind as well as their partners in crime, angel Xaphan and Morieshal destined to become legends. This is the tale of their youth and innocence. LEGENDS OF DESTINY volume 4 - 04 is taking place before the events of Prologue of Destiny, The Book of Elves, and Whisper of Destiny. This is LEGENDS OF DESTINY.

R

MidLife Crisis is a common theme for each of us as we reach the threshold. As a man, as a woman, why is it that half of the marriages end up in recall? If anything else would have half those rates of failure, the lawsuits would be raining. Where are the flaws, the traps? Love is strong and pure, why is marriage not the reflection of that? Those are all hard questions to ask with little or no answers. Dr. Bak is sharing his reflections and findings as he reached himself the WALL OF MARRIAGE. This is a matter that affects all of our lives. It is time for some answers.

THE GREAT PAUSE was a reboot of all the systems of society. Many outdated systems will not make it back. The Dental Industry is a needed one, it has laid on complacency for far too long. In an age where expertise is global and democratized and can be replaced with technologies and artificial intelligence, the REBOOT will force, not just an update, but an operating system replacement and a firmware upgrade. First, they saved their industry with THE ALPHAS INITIATIVE, sharing their knowledge and vision freely to all the world's dental industry. With the OUELLETTE INITIATIVE, they bought some time for all the dental clinics to resume and adjust. The warning has been given, the clock is now ticking. who will prevail and prosper and who will be left behind, outdated and obsolete?

RISING -062
TO WIN MORE THAN YOU ARE AFRAID TO LOSE
BY Dr. BAK NGUYEN

In RISING, TO WIN MORE TAN YOU ARE AFRAID TO LOSE, Dr. Bak is breaking down the strategy to success to all, not only those wearing white coats and scrubs. More than his previous book (SUCCESS IS A CHOICE), this one is covering most of the aspects of getting to the next level, psychologically, socially, and financially. Rising is broken down into three key strategies: Financial Leverage - Compressing time - Always being in control. Presented by MILLION DOLLAR MINDSET, the book is covering more than the ways to create wealth, but also how to reach happiness and live a life without regrets. Dr. Bak the CEO and founder of Mdex & Co, a company with the promise of reforming the whole dental industry for the better. He wrote more than 60 books within 30 months as he is sharing his experiences, secrets, and wisdom.

S

SELFMADE -036
GRATITUDE AND HUMILITY
BY Dr. BAK NGUYEN

This is the story of Dr. Bak, an artist who became a dentist, a dentist who became an Entrepreneur, an Entrepreneur who is seeking to save an entire industry. In his free time, Dr. Bak managed to write 37 books and is a contender for 3 world records to be confirmed. Businessman and visionary, his views and philosophy are ahead of our time. This is his 37th book. In SELFMADE, Dr. Bak is answering the questions most entrepreneurs want to know, the HOWTO and the secret recipes, not just to succeed, but to keep going no matter what! SELFMADE is the perfect read for any entrepreneurs, novices, and veterans.

SHORTCUT vol. 1 - HEALING 093
BY Dr. BAK NGUYEN

In SHORTCUT 408 HEALING QUOTES, Dr. Bak revisits and compiles his journey of healing and growing. Just like anyone, he was moulded and shaped by Conformity and Society to the point of blending and melting. Walking his journey of healing, he rediscovers himself and found his true calling. And once whole with himself and with the Universe, Dr. Bak found his powers. In SHORTCUT 408 HEALING QUOTES, you have a quick and easy way to surf his mindsets and what allowed him to heal, to find back his voice and wings, and to walk his destiny. You too are walking your Quest of Identity. That one is mainly a journey of healing. May you find yours and your powers.

SHORTCUT vol. 2 - GROWING 094
BY Dr. BAK NGUYEN

In SHORTCUT 408 GROWTH QUOTES, Dr. Bak is compiling his library of books about personal growth and self-improvement. More than a motivational book, more than a compilation of knowledge, Dr. Bak is sharing the mindsets upon which he found his power to achieve and to overachieve. We all have our powers, only they were muted and forgotten as we were forged by Conformity and Society. After the healing process, walking your Quest of Identity, the Quest for your growth and God-given power is next to lead you to walk your Destiny.

SHORTCUT vol. 3 - LEADERSHIP 095
BY Dr. BAK NGUYEN

In SHORTCUT 365 LEADERSHIP QUOTES, Dr. Bak is compiling his library of books about leadership and ambition. Yes, the ambition is to find your worth and to make the world a better place for all of us. If the 3rd volume of SHORTCUT is mainly a motivational compilation, it also holds the secrets and mindsets to influence and leadership. If you were looking to walk your legend and impact the world, you are walking a lonely path. You might on your own, but it does not have to be harder than it is. As we all have your unique challenges, the key to victory is often found in the same place, your heart. And here are 365 shortcuts to keep you believing and to attract more people to you as you are growing into a true leader.

SHORTCUT vol. 4 - CONFIDENCE -096
BY Dr. BAK NGUYEN

SHORTCUT 518 CONFIDENCE QUOTES, is the most voluminous compilation of Dr. Bak's quotes. To heal was the first step. To grow and find your powers came next. As you are walking your personal legend, Confidence is both your sword and armour to conquer your Destiny and overcome all of the challenges on your way. In SHORTCUT volume four, Dr. Bak comprises all his mindsets and wisdom to ease your ascension. Confidence is not something one is simply born with, but something to nurture, grow, and master. Some will have the chance to be raised by people empowering Confidence, others will have to heal from Conformity to grow their confidence. It does not matter, only once Confident, can one stand tall and see clearly the horizon.

SHORTCUT vol. 5- SUCCESS -097
BY Dr. BAK NGUYEN

Success is not a destination but a journey and a side effect. While no map can lead you to success, the right mindset will forge your own success, the one without medals nor labels. If you are looking to walk your legend, to be successful is merely the beginning. Actually, being successful is often a side effect of the mindsets and actions that you took, you provoked. In SHORTCUT 317 SUCCESS QUOTES, Dr. Bak is revisiting his journey, breaking down what led him to be successful despite the odds stacked against him. As success is the consequence of mindsets, choices, and actions, it can be duplicated over and over again, one just needs to master the mindsets first.

SHORTCUT vol. 6- POWER -098
BY Dr. BAK NGUYEN

That's the kind of power that you will discover within this journey. Power is a tool, a leverage. Well used, it will lead to great achievements. Misused, it will be your downfall. If a sword sometimes has 2 edges, Power is a sword with no handle and multiple edges. You have been warned. In SHORTCUT 376 POWER QUOTES, Dr. Bak is compiling all the powers he found and mastered walking his own legend. If the first power was Confidence, very quickly, Dr. Bak realized that Confidence was the key to many, many more powers. Where to find them, how to yield them, and how to leverage these powers is the essence of the 6th volume of SHORTCUT.

SHORTCUT vol. 7- HAPPINESS -099
BY Dr. BAK NGUYEN

We were all born happy and then, somehow, we lost our ways and forgot our ways home. Is this the real tragedy behind the lost paradise myth? If we were happy once, we can trust our hearts to find our way home, once more. This is the journey of the 7th volume of the SHORTCUT series. In

SHORTCUT 306 HAPPINESS QUOTES, Dr. Bak is revisiting and compiling all the secrets and mindsets leading to happiness. Happiness is not just a destination but a shrine for Confidence and a safe place to regroup, to heal, to grow. We each have our own happiness. What you will learn here is where to find yours and, more importantly, how to leverage you to ease the journey ahead, because happiness is not your final destination. It can be the key to your legend.

SHORTCUT vol. 8- DOCTORS -100
BY Dr. BAK NGUYEN

If healing was the first step to your destiny and powers, there is a science to healing. Those with that science are doctors, the healers of the world. In India, healers are second only to the Gods! In SHORTCUT 170 DOCTOR QUOTES, Dr. Bak is dedicating the 8th volume of the series to his peers, doctors, from all around the world. Doctors too, have to walk their Quest of Identity, to heal from their pain and to walk their legend. Doctors need to heal and rejuvenate to keep healing the world. If healing is their science, in SHORTCUT, they will access the power of leveraging.

SUCCESS IS A CHOICE -060
BLUEPRINTS FOR HEALTH PROFESSIONALS
BY Dr. BAK NGUYEN

In SUCCESS IS A CHOICE, FINANCIAL MILLIONAIRE BLUEPRINTS FOR HEALTH PROFESSIONALS, Dr. Bak is breaking down the strategy to success for all those wearing white coats and scrubs: doctors, dentists, pharmacists, chiropractors, nurses, etc. Success is broken down into three key strategies: Financial Leverage - Compressing time - Always being in control. Presented by MILLION DOLLAR MINDSET, the book is covering more than the ways to create wealth, but also how to reach happiness and live a life without regrets. Dr. Bak is a successful cosmetic dentist with nearly 20 years of experience. He founded Mdex & Co, a company with the promise of reforming the whole dental industry for the better. While doing so, he discovered a passion for writing and for sharing. Multiple times World Record, Dr. Bak is writing a book every 2 weeks for the last 30 months. This is his 60th book, and he is still practicing. How he does it, is what he is sharing with us, SUCCESS, HAPPINESS, and mostly FREEDOM to all Health Professionals.

SYMPHONY OF SKILLS -001
BY Dr. BAK NGUYEN

You will enlighten the world with your potential. I can't wait to see all the differences that you will have in our world. Remember that power comes with responsibility. We can feel in his presence, a genuine force, a depth of energy, confidence, innocence, courage, and intelligence. Bak is always looking for answers, morning and night, he wants to understand the why and the why not. This book is the essence of the man. Dr. Bak is a force of nature who bears proudly his title eHappy. The

431

man never ceases smiling and spreading his good vibe wherever he passes. He is not trapped in the nostalgia of the past nor the satisfaction of the present, he embodies the joy of what's possible, and what's to come. The more we read, the more we share, and we live. That is Bak, he charms us to evolve and to share his points of view, and before we know it, we are walking by his side, a journey we never saw coming.

T

THE 90 DAYS CHALLENGE -061
BY Dr. BAK NGUYEN

THE 90 DAYS CHALLENGE, is Dr. Bak's journey into the unknown. Overachiever writing 2 books a month on average, for the last 30 months, ambitious CEO, Industries' Disruptor, Dr. Bak seems to have success in everything he touches. Everything except the control of his weight. For nearly 20 years, he struggles with an overweight problem. Every time he scored big, he added on a little more weight. Well, this time, he exposes himself out there, in real-time and without filter, accepting the challenge of his brother-in-law, DON VO to lose 45 pounds within 90 days. That's half a pound a day, for three months. He will have to do so while keeping all of his other challenges on track, writing books at a world record pace, leading the dental industry into the new ERA, and keep seeing his patients. Undoubtedly entertaining, this is the journey of an ALPHA who simply won't give up. But this time, nothing is sure.

THE BOOK OF ANGELS -134
BY Dr. BAK NGUYEN & WILLIAM BAK

LEGENDS OF DESTINY, THE BOOK OF ANGELS is the Annals of the Angels of the Legends of Destiny. This book is the origin story and the fate of each of the angels and archangels from this epic fresque. As the worlds are clashing and the Gods are out of control, Ethem, the primal force created the angels to balance the forces of the universe. These are the stories of the guardians of balance, the wings of justice, and the tragedies of power and its corruption. Follow Angel Lord Adrian,

Archangel Mikael, Hermes, and Lucifer from their fights to their rise and demise. Follow the adventure of Angels Eto, Ethel, Jardoo; follow the rise of Dark Angels Anak, Felice, or Hesdielle. Choose your faction, Archangel, Angels, Dark Angels, Guild, Phantoms, bionics, or hybrid, you will each time be amazed. Caught between the Gods, the Titans, the demons, the elves, the orcs, the humans, and everything in between, the Angels bear the heavy responsibility of balancing life and creation. These are their legends.

THE BOOK OF LEGENDS -024
BY Dr. BAK NGUYEN & WILLIAM BAK

The Book of Legends vol. 1 is the story behind the world record of Dr. Bak and his son, William Bak. All Dr. Bak had in mind was to keep his promise of writing a book with his son. They ended up writing 8 children's books within a month, scoring a new world record. William is also the youngest author having published in two languages. Those are world records waiting to be confirmed. History will say: to celebrate a first world record (writing 15 books / 15 months), for the love of his son, he will have scored a second world record: to write 8 books within a month! THE BOOK OF LEGENDS vol. 1 This is both a magical journey for both a father and a son looking to connect and find themselves. Join Dr. Bak and William Bak in their journey and their love for Life!

THE BOOK OF LEGENDS 2 -041
BY Dr. BAK NGUYEN & WILLIAM BAK

THE BOOK OF LEGENDS vol. 2 is the sequel of "CINDERELLA" but a true story between a father and his son. Together they have discovered a bond and a way to connect. The first BOOK OF LEGENDS covered the time of the first four books they wrote together within a month. The second BOOK OF LEGENDS is covering what happened after the curtains dropped, and what happened after reality kicked back in. If the first volume was about a fairy tale in vacation time, the second volume is about making it last in real Life. Share their journey and their love of Life!

THE BOOK OF LEGENDS 3 -086
THE END OF THE INNOCENCE AGE
BY Dr. BAK NGUYEN & WILLIAM BAK

THE BOOK OF LEGENDS 3 is a long work extending to almost 3 years. If the shocking duo known as Dr. Bak and prodigy William Bak has marked the imaginary writing world record upon world record, the story is not all pink. After the franchise of the CHICKEN BOOKS, William, now in his pre-teen years, wants to move away from the chicken tales. After 22 chicken books, a break is well deserved. that said, what is next? Both father and son thought that if they could do it once easily, they could do it again! They couldn't be any further from the truth. For 2 years, they were stuck in the quest for their next franchise of books. THE BOOK OF LEGENDS 3 started right around the end of the chicken franchise and would have ended with a failure if the book was to be released on time, the holiday season of that year. It took the duo another year to complete their story to add the last chapters of this book, hoping to end with a happy ending. Unfortunately, not all story ends the way we wish... this is the dark tome of the series, where the imagination got eclipsed. Follow William and Dr. Bak in their fight to keep the magic and connection alive.

THE CONFESSION OF A LAZY OVERACHIEVER -089
REINVENT YOURSELF FROM ANY CRISIS
BY Dr. BAK NGUYEN

In THE CONFESSION OF A LAZY OVERACHIEVER, Dr. Bak is opening up to his new marketing officer, Jamie, fresh out of school. She is young, full of energy, and looking to chill and still have it all. True to his character, Dr. Bak is giving Jamie some leeway to redefine Dr. Bak's brand to her demographic, the Millennials. This journey is about Dr. Bak satisfying the Millennials and answering their true questions in life. A rebel himself, his ambition to change the world started back on campus, some 25 years ago... then, life caught up with him. It took Dr. Bak 20 years to shake down the burdens of life, spread his wings free from Conformity, and start Overachieving. Doctor, CEO, and world record author, here is what Dr. Bak would have loved to know 25 years ago as was still on campus. In a word, this is cheating your way to success and freedom. And yes, it is possible. Success, Money, and Freedom, they all start with a mindset and the awareness of Time. Welcome to the Alphas.

THE ENERGY FORMULA -053
BY Dr. BAK NGUYEN

THE ENERGY FORMULA is a book dedicated to helping each individual to find the means to reach their purpose and goal in Life. Dr. Bak is a philosopher, a strategist, a business, an artist, and a dentist, how does he do all of that? He is doing so while mentoring proteges and leading the modernization of an entire industry. Until now, Momentum and Speed were the powers that he was building on and from. But those powers come from somewhere too. From a guide of our Quest of Identity, he became an ally in everyone's journey for happiness. THE ENERGY FORMULA is the book revealing step by step, the logic of building the right mindset and the way to ABUNDANCE and HAPPINESS, universally. It is not just a HOW TO book, but one that will change your life and guide you to the path of ABUNDANCE.

THE MODERN WOMAN 070
TO HAVE IT HAVE WITH NO SACRIFICE
BY Dr. BAK NGUYEN & Dr. EMILY LETRAN

In THE MODERN WOMAN: TO HAVE IT ALL WITH NO SACRIFICE, Dr. Bak joins forces with Dr. Emily Letran to empower all women to fulfill their desires, goals, and ambition. Both overachievers going against the odds, they are sharing their experience and wisdom to help all women to find confidence and support to redefine their lives. Dr. Emily Letran is a doctor in dentistry, an entrepreneur, author, and CERTIFIED HIGH-PERFORMANCE coach. For an Asian woman, she made it through the norms and the red tapes to find her voice. As she learnt and grew with mentors, today she is sharing her secret with the energy that will motivate all of the female genders to stand for what they deserve. Alpha doctor, Bak is joining his voice and perspective since this is not about gender equality, but about personal empowerment and the quest of Identity of each, man and woman. Once more, Dr. Bak is bringing LEVERAGE and REASON to the new social deal between man and woman. This is not about gender, but about confidence.

THE POWER BEHIND THE ALPHA 008
BY TRANIE VO & Dr. BAK NGUYEN

It's been said by a "great man" that "We are born alone and we die alone." Both men and women proudly repeat those words as wisdom since. I apologize in advance, but what a fat LIE! That's what I learnt and discovered in life since my mind and heart got liberated from the burden of scars and the ladders of society. I can have it all, not all at the same time, but I can have everything I put my mind and heart into. Actually, it is not completely true. I can have most of what I and Tranie put our minds into. Together, when we feel like one, there isn't much out of our reach. If I'm the mind, she's the heart; if I'm the Will, she's the means. Synergy is the core of our power. Tranie's aim is always Happiness. In Tranie's definition of life, there are no justifications, no excuses, no tomorrow. For Tranie, Happiness is measured by the minutes of every single day. This is why she's so strong and can heal people around her. That may also be why she doesn't need to talk much, since talking about the past or the future is, in her mind, dimming down the magic of the present, the Now. We both respect and appreciate that we are the whole balancing each other's equation of life, of love, of success. I was the plus and the minus, then I became the multiplication factor and grew into the exponential. And how is Tranie evolving in all of this? She is and always will be the balance. If anything, she is the equal sign of each equation.

THE POWER OF Dr. -066
THE MODERN TITLE OF NOBILITY
BY Dr. BAK NGUYEN, Dr. PAVEL KRASTEV AND COLLABORATORS

In THE POWER OF Dr., independent thinkers mean to exchange ideas. An idea can be very powerful if supported by a great work ethic. Work ethic, isn't that the main fabric of our white coats, scrubs, and title? In an era post-COVID where everything has been rebooted and that's the healthcare industry is facing its own fate: to evolve or to be replaced, Dr. Bak and Dr. Pavel reveal the source of their power and their playbook to move forward, ahead. The power we all hold is our resilience and discipline. We put that for years at the service of our profession, from a surgical perspective. Now, we can harness that same power to rewrite the rules, the industry, and our future. Post-COVID, the rules are being rewritten, will you be part of the team or left behind? "You can be in control!" More than personal growth and a motivational book, THE POWER OF Dr. is an awakening call to the doctor you look at when you graduate, with hope, with honour, with determination.

THE POWER OF YES -010
VOLUME ONE: IMPACT
BY Dr. BAK NGUYEN

In THE POWER OF YES, Dr. Bak is sharing his journey, opening up and embracing the world, one day at a time, one task at a time, one wish at a time. Far from a dare, saying YES allowed Dr. Bak to rewrite his mindset and break all the boundaries. This book is not one written in a few days or weeks, but the accumulation of a journey for 12 months. The journey started as Dr. Bak said YES to his producer to go on stage and speak… That YES opened a world of possibilities. Dr. Bak embraced each and every one of them. 12 months later, he is celebrating the new world record of writing 9 books written over a period of 12 months. To him, it will be a miss, missing the 12 on 12 mark. To the rest of the world, they just saw the birth of a force of nature, the Alpha force. THE POWER OF YES is comprised of all the introductions of the adult books written by Dr. Bak within the first 12 months. Chapter by chapter, you can walk in his footstep seeing and smelling what he has. This is reality-literature with a twist of POWER. THE POWER OF YES! Discover your potential and your power. This is the POWER OF YES, volume one. Welcome to the Alphas.

THE POWER OF YES 2 -037
VOLUME TWO: SHAPELESS
BY Dr. BAK NGUYEN

In THE POWER OF YES, volume 2, Dr. Bak is continuing his journey, discovering his powers and influence. After 12 months of embracing the world by saying YES, he rose as an emerging force:

he's been recognized as an INDUSTRIES DISRUPTOR, got nominated ERNST AND YOUNG ENTREPRENEUR OF THE YEAR, wrote 9 books within 12 months while launching the most ambitious private endeavour to reform his own industry, the dental field. Contender too many WORLD RECORDS, Dr. Bak is doing all of that in parallel. And yes, he is sleeping his nights and yes, he is writing his book himself, from the screen of his iPhone! Far from satisfied, Dr. Bak missed the mark of writing 12 books within 12 months. While everything is taking shape, everything could also crumble down at each turn. Now that Dr. Bak understands his powers, he is looking to test them and push them to their limits, looking to keep scoring world records while materializing his vision and enterprises. This is the awakening of a Force of Nature looking to change the world for the better while having fun sharing. Welcome to the Alphas.

THE POWER OF YES 3 046
VOLUME THREE: LIMITLESS
BY Dr. BAK NGUYEN

In THE POWER OF YES, volume 3, the journey of Dr. Bak continues where the last volume left, in front of 300 plus people showing up to his first solo event, a Dr. Bak's event. On stage and in this book, Dr. Bak reveals how 12 months of saying YES to everything changed his life... actually, it was 18 months. From a dentist looking to change the world from a dental chair into a multiple times world record author, the journey of openness is a rendezvous with Fate. Dr. Bak is sharing almost in real-time his journey, and experiences, but above all, his feelings, doubts, and comebacks. From one book to the next, from one journey to the next, follow the adventure of a man looking to find his name, his worth, and his place in the world. Doing so, he is touching people Doing so, he is touching people and initiating their rise. Are you ready for more? Are you ready to meet your Fate and Destiny? Welcome to the Alphas.

THE POWER OF YES 4 087
VOLUME FOUR: RISING
BY Dr. BAK NGUYEN

In THE POWER OF YES, volume 4, the journey continues days after where the last volume left. After setting the new world record of writing 48 books within 24 months, Dr. Bak is not ready to stop. As volume one covers 12 months of journey, volume 2 covers 6 months. Well, volume 3 covers 4 months. The speed is building up and increasing, steadily. This is volume 4, RISING, after breaking the sound barrier. Dr. Bak has reached a state where he is above most resistance and friction, he is now in a universe of his own, discovering his powers as he walks his journeys. This is no fiction story or wishful thinking, THE POWER OF YES is the journey of Dr. Bak, from one world record to the next, from one book to the next. You too can walk your own legend, you just need to listen to your innersole and open up to the opportunity. May you get inspiration from the legendary journey of Dr. Bak and find your own Destiny. Welcome to the Alphas.

THE RISE OF THE UNICORN -038
BY Dr. BAK NGUYEN & Dr. JEAN DE SERRES

In THE RISE OF THE UNICORN, Dr. Bak is joining forces with his friend and mentor, Dr. Jean De Serres. Together both men had many achievements in their respective industries, but the advent of eHappyPedia, THE RISE OF THE UNICORN is a personal project dear to both of them: the QUEST OF HAPPINESS and its empowerment. This book is a special one since you are witnessing the conversation between two entrepreneurs looking to change the world by building unique tools and media. Just like any enterprise, the ride is never a smooth one in the park on a beautiful day. But this is about eHappyPedia, it is about happiness, right? So it will happen and with a smile attached to it! The unique value of this book is that you are sharing the ups and downs of the launch of a Unicorn, not just the glory of the fame, but also the doubts and challenges along the way. May it inspire you on your own journey to success and happiness.

THE RISE OF THE UNICORN 2 -076
eHappyPedia
BY Dr. BAK NGUYEN & Dr. JEAN DE SERRES

This is 2 years after starting the first tome. Dr. Bak's brand is picking up, between the accumulation of records and recognition. eHappyPedia is now hot for a comeback. In THE RISE OF THE UNICORN 2, Dr. Bak is retracing and addressing each of Dr. Jean De Serres' concerns about the weakness of the first version of eHappyPedia and the eHappy movement. This is the sort of creation and a UNICORN both in finance and in psychology. Never before, have you assisted in such a daily and decision-making process of a world phenomenon and of a company. Dr. Bak and Dr. De Serres are literally using the process of writing this series of books to plan and brainstorm the birth of a bluechip. More than an intriguing story, this is the journey of 2 experienced entrepreneurs changing the world.

THE U.A.X STORY -072
THE ULTIMATE AUDIO EXPERIENCE
BY Dr. BAK NGUYEN

This is the story of the ULTIMATE AUDIO EXPERIENCE, U.A.X. Follow Dr. Bak's footsteps in how he invented a new way to read and learn. Dr. Bak brings his experience as a movie producer and a director to elevate the reading experience to another level with entertaining value and make it accessible to everyone, auditive, and visual people alike. After three years plus of research and development, and countless hours of trials and errors, Dr. Bak finally solved his puzzle: having written more than 1.1 million words. The irony is that he does not like to read, he likes audiobooks! U.A.X. finally allowed the opening of Dr. Bak's entire library to a new genre and media. U.A.X. is the new way to learn and enjoy Audiobooks. Made to be entertaining while keeping the self-educational value of a book, U.A.X. will appeal to both auditive and visual people. U.A.X. is the blockbuster of Audiobooks. The format has already been approved by iTunes, Amazon, Spotify, and all major platforms for global distribution and streaming.

THE VACCINE -077
BY Dr. BAK NGUYEN & WILLIAM BAK

In THE VACCINE, A TALE OF SPIES AND ALIENS, Dr. Bak reprises his role as mentor to William, his 10-year-old son, both as co-author and as doctor. William is living through the COVID war and has accumulated many, many questions. That morning, they got out all at once. From a conversation between father and son, Dr. Bak is making science into words keeping the interest of his son on a Saturday morning in bed. William is not just an audience, he is responsible to map the field with his questions. What started as a morning conversation between father and son, became within the next hour, a great project, their 23rd book together. Learn about the virus, and vaccination while entertaining your kids.

TIMING - TIME MANAGEMENT ON STEROIDS -074
BY Dr. BAK NGUYEN & WILLIAM BAK

In TIMING, TIME MANAGEMENT ON STEROIDS, Dr. Bak is sharing his secret to keep overachieving, and overdelivering while raising the bar higher and higher. We all have 24 hours in a day, so how can some do so much more than others? Dr. Bak is not only sharing his secrets and mindset about time and efficiency, he is literally living his own words as this book is written within his last sprint to set the next world record of writing 100 books within 4 years, with only 31 days to go. With 8 books to write in 31 days, that's a little less than 4 days per book! Share the journey of a man surfing the change and looking to see where is the limit of the human mind, writing. In the meantime, understand his leverage, mindset, and secrets to challenge your own limits and dreams.

TO OVERACHIEVE EVERYTHING BEING LAZY -090
CHEAT YOUR WAY TO SUCCESS
BY Dr. BAK NGUYEN

In TO OVERACHIEVE EVERYTHING BEING LAZY, Dr. Bak retakes his role talking to the millennials, the next generation. If in the first tome of the series LAZY, Dr. Bak addresses the general audience of millennials, especially young women, he is dedicating this tome to the ALPHA amongst the millennials, those aiming for the moon and looking, not only to be happy but to change the world. This is not another take on how to cheat your way to success or how to leverage laziness, but this is the recipe to build overachievers and rainmakers. For the young leaders with ambitions and talent, understanding TIME and ENERGY are crucial from your first steps in writing your our legend. If Dr. Bak had the chance to do it all over again, this is how he would do it! Welcome to the Alphas.

TORNADO -067
FORCE OF CHANGE
BY Dr. BAK NGUYEN

In TORNADO - FORCE OF CHANGE Dr. Bak is writing solo. In the midst of the COVID war, change is not a good intention anymore. Change, constant change has become a new reality, a new norm. From somebody who holds the title of Industries' Disruptor, how does he yield change to stay in control? Well, the changes from the COVID war are constant fear and much loss of individual liberty. Some can endure the change, some will ride it. Dr. Bak is sharing his angle of navigating the changes, yielding the improvisations, and to reinvent the goals, the means to stay relevant. From fighting to keep his companies Dr. Bak went on to let go of the uncontrollable to embrace the opportunity, he reinvented himself to ride the change and create opportunities from an unprecedented crisis. This is the story of a man refusing to kneel and accept defeat, smiling back at faith to find leverage and hope.

TOUCHSTONE -073
LEVERAGING TODAY'S PSYCHOLOGICAL SMOG
BY Dr. BAK NGUYEN & Dr. KEN SEROTA

TOUCHSTONE, LEVERAGING TODAY'S PSYCHOLOGICAL SMOG is mapping to navigate and thrive in today's high and constant stress environment. After 40 years in practice, Dr. Serota is concerned about the evolution of the career of health care professionals and the never-ending level of stress. What is stress, and what are its effects, damages, and symptoms? If COVID-19 revealed to the world that we are fragile, it also revealed most of the broken and the flaws of our system. For now a century, dentistry has been a champion in depression, Drug addiction, and suicide rates, and the curve is far from flattening. Dr. Bak is sharing his perspective and experience dealing with stress and how to leverage it into a constructive force. From the stress of a doctor with no right to failure to the stress of an entrepreneur never knowing the future, Dr. Bak is sharing his way to use stress as leverage.

WHISPER OF DARKNESS -135
BY Dr. BAK NGUYEN & WILLIAM BAK

WHISPER OF DARKNESS is the 3rd volume of LEGENDS OF DESTINY. This time, the story is set at the celestial level, as the war between the angels is raging. After Adrian's ascension to power, the dissident angels left. Some stay isolated as Archangel Anton and Lucifer and will be known as the

Errants. Others will regroup and organize. Heaven calls them the Dark Angels, those no more within the light of Heaven. Between the raids to put down the Gods out of control, Heaven is also sending squadrons of Angels to hunt down the dissidents with more or less success. This is the story of angels Ethel and Eto, as they are sent on a recognition mission to uncover the whereabouts of Kohël, a dissident angel, now known as Dali, the God of the Wind. Both junior angels looking to prove their worth to Heaven, the Council of Angels, and their Angel Lord, Adrian. Well, they are not the only ones looking to make their mark, as Hasdielle, a Dark Angel, is also looking to prove Heaven weak and wrong! Follow the legend of Ethel and Eto in WHISPER OF DARKNESS, the 3rd volume of LEGENDS OF DESTINY.

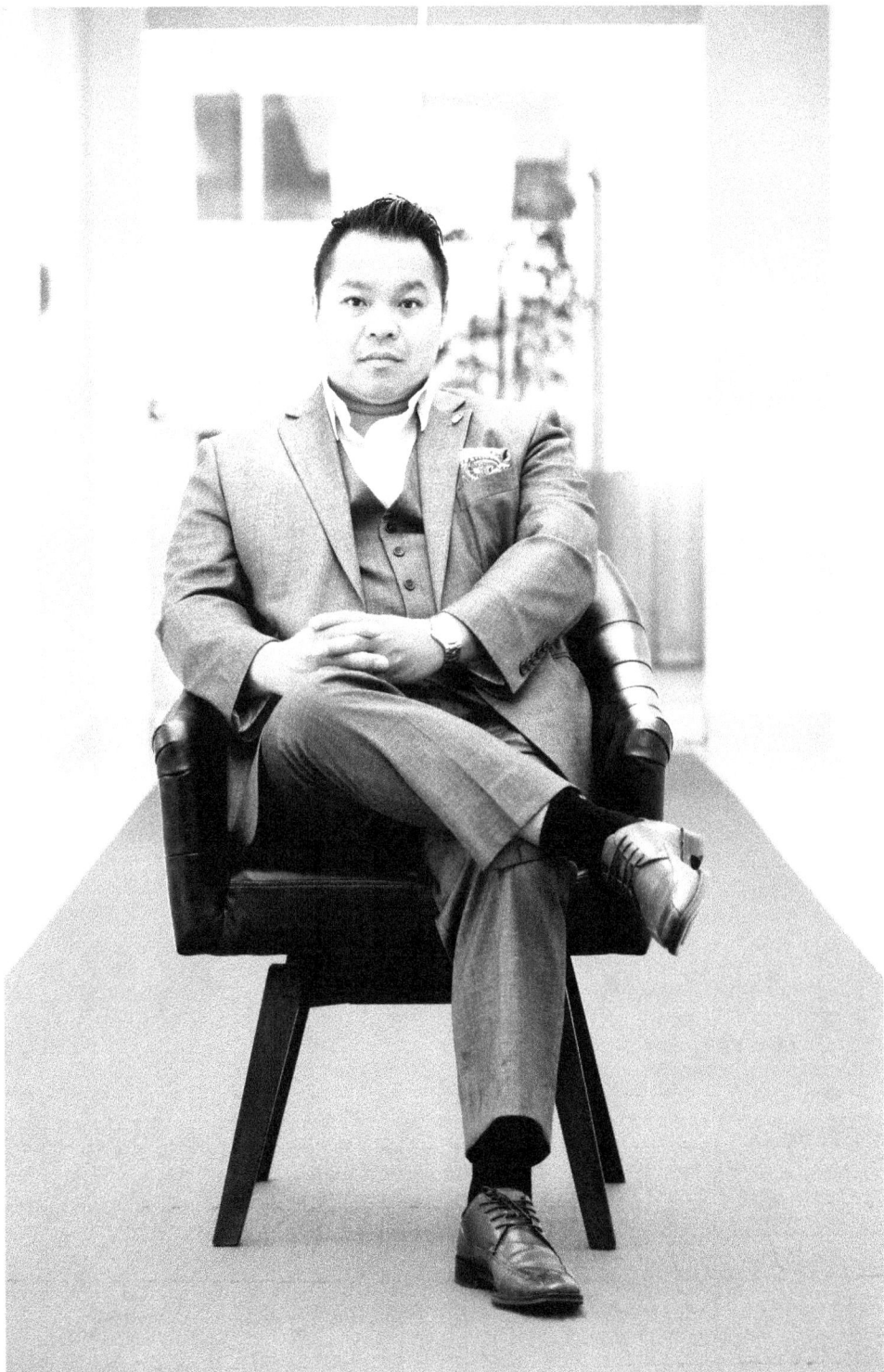

ABOUT THE AUTHORS

From Canada ♦, **Dr. BAK NGUYEN**, Nominee Ernst and Young Entrepreneur of the year, Grand Homage Lys DIVERSITY, LinkedIn & TownHall Achiever of the year and TOP 100 Doctors 2021. In 2023, he made the CREA GLOBAL AWARD list. Dr. Bak is a cosmetic dentist, CEO and founder of Mdex & Co. His company is revolutionizing the dental field.

Speaker and motivator, he holds the world record of writing 120 books in 5 years accumulating many world records (to be officialized). Before that, he held the world record of writing 9 books over 12 months, then, 15 books within 15 months to set the bar even higher with the world record of 36 books written within 18 months + 1 week.

By his second author anniversary, he scored his new landmark world record of 48 books within 24 months. And then 72 books in 36 months. By the 4th anniversary, Dr. Bak scored his usual landmark of writing 96 books over 48 months, but he pushed even further, scoring also the landmark world record of 100 books written within 4 years and then, 120 books written in 5 years! His books are covering:

ENTREPRENEURSHIP - LEADERSHIP - QUEST OF IDENTITY - DENTISTRY AND MEDICINE - PARENTING - CHILDREN BOOKS - PHILOSOPHY

In 2003, he founded Mdex, a dental company upon which in 2018, he launched the most ambitious private endeavour to reform the dental industry, Canada-wide. Philosopher, he has close to his heart the quest of happiness of the people surrounding him, patients and colleagues alike. In 2020, he launched an International collaborative initiative named **THE ALPHAS** to share knowledge and for Entrepreneurs and Doctors to thrive through the Greatest Pandemic and Economic depression of our time.

In 2016, he co-found with Tranie Vo, Emotive World Incorporated, a tech research company to use technology to empower happiness and sharing. U.A.X. the ultimate audio experience is the landmark project on which the team is advancing, utilizing the technics of the movie industry and the advancement in ARTIFICIAL INTELLIGENCE to save the book industry and upgrade the continuing education space.

These projects have allowed Dr. Nguyen to attract interest from the international and diplomatic community and he is now the centre of a global discussion on the wellbeing and the future of the health profession. It is in that matter that he shares his thoughts and encourages the health community to share their own stories. Motivational speaker and serial entrepreneur, philosopher and author, in his own words, Dr. Nguyen describes himself as a dentist by circumstances, an entrepreneur by nature and a communicator by passion. He also holds recognitions from the Canadian Parliament and the Canadian Senate.

From the USA 🇺🇸, **Dr. PAUL DOMINIQUE**, is a paediatric dentist, entrepreneur and investor. He's a graduate of the National University of Ireland, where he earned a Bachelor of Science degree in cell biology and molecular genetics. He completed his dental degree at the University of Kentucky and his specialty training in paediatrics at the Eastman Institute for Oral Health, University of Rochester, NY. Dr. Dominique served as an assistant professor in public health at the University of Kentucky, division of oral health science. During his tenure, he headed and improved a novel mobile program that successfully addresses access to care issues for children in Central and Western Kentucky. Dr. Dominique is also an entrepreneur having acquired and consolidated a small group of practices growing from less than 700K to over 2.4 Million EBITDA in under 24 months. Dr. Dominique has been angel investing for the past decade, investing across a diverse group of platforms such as equity crowdfunding, psychedelic medicine, real estate and teledentistry. He currently serves as a board advisory member to the Teledentists and Revere Partners, the first venture fund dedicated to oral health. He's currently involved in a project that is exploring the use of blockchain technology and NFTs to help improve access to dental care.

From the USA 🇺🇸, **Dr. RICHARD SIMPSON**, DMD, is a board-certified paediatric dentist in private practice and a veteran with 15 years of military service. Dr. Simpson is a Diplomate in the American Board of Paediatric Dentistry, and a Fellow in The American College of Dentists, the International College of Dentists, and the American Academy of Pediatric Dentistry. He has held numerous health professional leadership positions and has experience in state and national cross-sector networking, telehealth/teledentistry, child advocacy, health disparities, policy, and advancing improved medical-dental integration and access to care. He is skilled in leadership, project design and implementation, advocacy, and inter-professional and public-private collaboration. He believes that telehealth is the integral to the future of dentistry and the oral health-overall healthcare paradigm. Dr Simpson is the Immediate Past-Chair of the Oral Health Coalition of Alabama, He serves as and has recently completed his tenure as the Chief Clinical Officer for Holland Healthcare, an international telehealth oral imaging innovator. Dr. Simpson is a member of the Advisory Boards of The TeleDentists and Soluria He and he serves as a Thought Leader and collaborator with TeethCloud, a global oral health initiative dedicated to reducing oral health inequities through technology and DI. Dr. Simpson was recently selected to the 2023 Class of the World's Top 100 Doctors by members of the Global Summits Institute.

From the USA 🇺🇸, **Dr. MARILYN SANDOR**, DDS, MS, is one of Southwest Florida's favourite paediatric dentists. She is highly experienced in her field, having founded her private practice, Naples Paediatric Dentistry in the beautiful community of Naples, Florida in 2001. Dr. Sandor is a successful business owner and an active member of her community. She is committed to educating her young patients on the importance of oral health and enjoys teaching children how to have healthy smiles for a lifetime. Dr. Sandor's paediatric-focused invention, Zooby prophy angles, inspired a full line of creative new products by Young Innovations, which have been bringing joy to dental patients around the world for over a decade. She is the founder and CEO of the GoodCheckup Corporation, a new software company that provides easily accessible and equitable platforms for dentists to expand their reach via a mobile-to-mobile, patent-pending, teledentistry solution. GoodCheckup's flagship products, GoodCheckup Patient and GoodCheckup Doctor are the first Cloud-based, comprehensive smartphone teledentistry applications created by a paediatric dentist specifically for paediatric dentistry.

From the USA 🇺🇸, **Dr. NIDHI TANEJA**, DDS, MSD, is a board-certified paediatric dentist. She is an expert in seeing children with special needs and those with dental fear and anxiety. She wants no child to ever be scared of going to the dentist. Her unique behavior guidance and minimally invasive techniques, help children get through their dental visits with trust and confidence. After being in the conventional model of clinical dentistry which is heavily driven by procedures and surgical intervention, her goal is to help families and children experience dentistry without drills and fears. As a positive childhood advocate, she incorporates mindfulness-based principles in her practice for optimal oral and mental hygiene. She has been awarded 40 under 40 America's Best Dental Specialists, selected for Guiding Leaders program for Women Leadership and is actively involved in organized dentistry with theAmerican Dental Association and the American Academy of Paediatric Dentistry.

From GERMANY 🇩🇪, **Dr. AURORA ALVA**, DMD, is an American board-certified pediatric dentist, a member of the American College of Paediatric Dentists, and a diplomate of the American Board of Paediatric Dentists. She started her career by obtaining a Biology degree from Wellesley College in Wellesley, Massachusetts, where she graduated Cum Laude. During her time at Wellesley, she also had the opportunity to successfully complete courses at the Massachusetts Institute of Technology (MIT) and immersed herself in summer research projects at Harvard Medical School. She obtained various college stipends for her achievements such as from the Howard Hughes Medical Institute, and upon graduation, was one of the two recipients of the Wellesley College Graduate Fellowship Award. She obtained her dental degree and Paediatric Dentistry certificate from Tufts School of Dental Medicine in Boston, Massachusetts, in 2007 and 2009 respectively. Dr. Alva's pediatric dental professional career has been diverse. She has worked in private practice in Massachusetts, Texas and Georgia, participated in humanitarian dental missions in Honduras and Ecuador, worked as a pediatric dental contractor for the American Army in Germany, and worked in private practices in Munich, Germany. Dr. Aurora Alva holds professional licenses from the states of Georgia, Texas, Hawaii, California, Massachustetts and the region of Bavaria in Germany. She is an active member of the American Dental Association, the American Academy of Paediatric Dentists, and the American Board of Pediatric Dentists.

From EGYPT 🇪🇬, **Dr. NOUR AMMAR**, BDS, MS. She is a dedicated specialist in pediatric dentistry and dental public health hailing from Egypt. With an impressive educational background from Alexandria University's Faculty of Dentistry, including graduating top of her class in her bachelor's degree and master's degree, Dr. Ammar has already achieved so much in her field. She has served as a teaching assistant at the same institution for five years, demonstrating her passion for sharing knowledge with others. In addition to her academic accomplishments, Dr. Ammar is also a Harvard alumnus and has participated in a clinical research program there. Her clinical work has earned her several distinguished awards, demonstrating her exceptional skills and commitment to improving patient outcomes. Currently pursuing a Ph.D. at the University of Munich in Germany, Dr. Ammar is committed to raising awareness and knowledge of oral health, particularly among parents and children. Her vision of improving access to dental care for underprivileged or remote populations is being realized through the development of an AI program that can assist primary healthcare centers in identifying different dental pathologies without the real-time presence of a specialist. With her passion for pediatric dentistry and dental public health, Dr. Nour Ammar is a true asset to her profession.

From PERU ▌▌, **Dr. AILIN CABRERA-MATTA**, DDS, MSc, Ph.D., is an associate professor at the Peruvian University Cayetano Heredia. In addition to being a pediatrician, she holds a master's degree in epidemiology, a master's degree in pediatric dentistry, and a doctorate in public health. Her primary interests lie in maternal and child health and the prevention of early childhood caries. She is focused on global health and public health, specifically in relation to children's oral health.

From ITALY ▌▌, **Dr. PIERLUIGI PELAGALLI**, DDS, obtained his degree in Dentistry and Dental Prosthetics from the University of Naples Federico II in 1990. He further specialized in Paediatric Dentistry at the University of L'Aquila and focused his training on periodontology, implantology, and prosthetics. Over the years, he has developed a keen interest in paediatric dentistry and new technologies. Dr. Paelagalli received his periodontal surgery and guided tissue regeneration specialization in 1992 from the Royal Dental School in Aarhus, directed by Professor T. Karring. He attended continuing dental education at New York University and various other specialization courses in Oral Surgery and Fixed Prosthesis. He is a student of Dr. Roberto Olivi for children's dentistry. Dr. Paelagalli has been a professor since 2017 at the Master "Fixed prosthesis on natural teeth and implants" at the University of Rome "La Sapienza." He founded the network "the children's dentist" in 2007, and he is interested in promoting the health of children's mouths. Dr. Pelagalli has published several works, including the classification of implant sites and related therapeutic indications, the advantages of using an Er:YAG laser in pedodontics surgery, Kids Cario Test, and Kids Digital Crown Technique. He is a member of various dental societies and is currently working as a freelancer in Rome.

From UNITED ARAB EMIRATES ▬, **Dr. PRRIYA PORWAL**, BDS, MSD, is a paediatric dentist practicing in Abu Dhabi since 2019. She has developed an interest in psychology and clinical hypnotherapy, which she applies to help manage anxiety and uncooperative behaviour of her patients. She has been awarded the Indian Health Professional Awards 2020 for Excellence in Pedodontics. She has been privileged to work with the team of Oncology department in Burjeel Medical City, Abu Dhabi, UAE; as a Specialist Pediatric Dentist, doing Full Mouth Rehabilitation for children requiring Bone Marrow Transplant. . Additionally, she has a strong passion for art, which plays a significant role in her life and influences her approach to dentistry.

UAX

ULTIMATE AUDIO EXPERIENCE

A new way to learn and enjoy Audiobooks. Made to be entertaining while keeping the self-educational value of a book, UAX will appeal to both auditive and visual people. UAX is the blockbuster of the Audiobooks.

UAX will cover most of Dr. Bak's books, and is now negotiating to bring more authors and more titles to the UAX concept. Now streaming on Spotify, Apple Music and available for download on all major music platforms. Give it a try today!

AMAZON - BARNES & NOBLE - APPLE BOOKS - KINDLE
SPOTIFY - APPLE MUSIC

FROM THE SAME AUTHOR
Dr. Bak Nguyen

www.Dr.BakNguyen.com

LEADERSHIP vol. 1 -121
CHANGING THE WORLD FROM A
DENTAL CHAIR

🏴 ALBANIA 🔵 BRAZIL 🍁 CANADA
🏳 HUNGARY 🇲🇾 MALAYSIA 🏴 SPAIN
🏳 USA

BY Dr. BAK NGUYEN, Dr. MAHSA KHAGHANI,
Dr. NAGY KATALIN, with guest authors Dr. PAUL
DOMINIQUE, Dr. PAUL OUELLETTE, Dr. GURIEN
DEMIRAQI, Dr. BENNETE FERNANDES, Dr.
SANDRA FABIANO, Dr. ARASH HAKHAMIAN
and Dr. MARILYN SANDOR

ALPHA DENTISTRY vol. 2 -127
IMPLANTOLOGY FAQ ASSEMBLED
EDITION

🏴 ALBANIA 🔵 BRAZIL 🍁 CANADA
🏳 INDIA 🇲🇾 MALAYSIA 🏴 PORTUGAL
🏴 SPAIN 🏳 USA

BY Dr. BAK NGUYEN, Dr. ÉRIC LACOSTE,
Dr. PREETINDER SINGH AHLUWALIA,
Dr. BENNETE FERNANDES, Dr. SANDRA
FABIANO, Dr. SANDEEP SINGH, Dr. ERIC
PULVER, Dr. RAQUEL ZITA GOMES, Dr. GURIEN
DEMIRAQI, Dr. MASHA KHAGHANI and
Dr. ARASH HAKHAMIAN

ALPHA DENTISTRY vol. 2 -128
IMPLANTOLOGY FAQ INTERNATIONAL
EDITION

🏳 ENGLISH 🏴 ALBANIAN 🍁 FRANÇAIS
🏴 GERMAN 🏳 HINDI 🏳 ITALIAN
🏳 KANNADA 🇲🇾 MALAY 🏴 MANDARIN
🏴 PORTUGUESE 🏴 SPANISH

BY Dr. BAK NGUYEN, Dr. ÉRIC LACOSTE,
Dr. PREETINDER SINGH AHLUWALIA,

Dr. BENNETE FERNANDES, Dr. SANDRA
FABIANO, Dr. SANDEEP SINGH, Dr. ERIC
PULVER, Dr. RAQUEL ZITA GOMES, Dr. GURIEN
DEMIRAQI, Dr. MASHA KHAGHANI and Dr.
ARASH HAKHAMIAN

ALPHA DENTISTRY vol. 3 -131
PAEDIATRIC DENTISTRY FAQ
ASSEMBLED EDITION

🍁 CANADA 🏴 EGYPT 🏴 GERMANY
🏳 ITALY 🏳 PERU 🏴 UNITED ARAB
EMIRATES 🏳 USA

BY Dr. BAK NGUYEN,
Dr. PAUL DOMINIQUE, Dr. RICHARD SIMPSON,
Dr. MARILYNE SANDOR, Dr. AURORA ALVA,
Dr. NOUR AMMAR, Dr. AILIN CABRERA-MATTA,
Dr. NIDHI TANEJA, Dr. PRRIYA PORWAL,
and Dr. PIERLUIGI PELAGALLI

ALPHA DENTISTRY vol. 3 -132
PAEDIATRIC DENTISTRY FAQ
INTERNATIONAL EDITION

🍁 CANADA 🏴 EGYPT 🏴 GERMANY
🏳 ITALY 🏳 PERU 🏴 UNITED ARAB
EMIRATES 🏳 USA

BY Dr. BAK NGUYEN,
Dr. PAUL DOMINIQUE, Dr. RICHARD SIMPSON,
Dr. MARILYNE SANDOR, Dr. AURORA ALVA,
Dr. NOUR AMMAR, Dr. AILIN CABRERA-MATTA,
Dr. NIDHI TANEJA, Dr. PRRIYA PORWAL,
and Dr. PIERLUIGI PELAGALLI

THE LAZY FRANCHISE

TEEN'S FICTION
with William Bak

SOCIETY

LEGENDS OF DESTINY

www.Dr.BakNguyen.com

UNLIMITED ACCESS
DR. BAK'S ENTIRE AUDIO LIBRARY

Since Dr. Bak set his new landmark world record of writing 100 books in 4 years, he is opening his entire audio library, audiobooks and UAX albums, exclusively to all VIP members for $9.99/month.

By becoming a VIP member, you will have access to all Dr. Bak's audiobooks and UAX albums. Those are the ones today bought at Apple Books, Audible, and in COMBO version at Amazon. The UAX albums are those streaming on Apple Music, Spotify, and Amazon Prime Music.

As a VIP, you will also have prime access to the audiobooks as soon as they are completed, hitting them before they reach the mainstream outlets. Get your membership today!

http://drbaknguyen.com/members

Welcome to the Alphas.

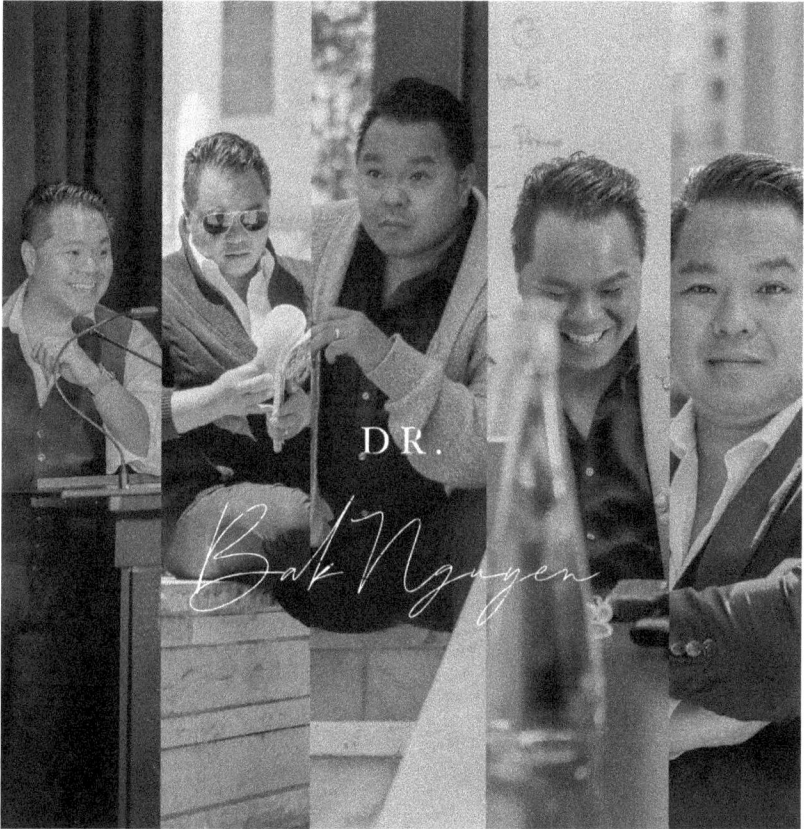

DR.

Bak Nguyen

www.ingramcontent.com/pod-product-compliance
Lightning Source LLC
Chambersburg PA
CBHW052100230326
41599CB00054B/3383

* 9 7 8 1 9 9 8 7 5 0 1 8 4 *